Dilemmas and Decision Making in Speech and Language Therapy

AF739713

This book presents a variety of dilemmas that highlight the breadth and complexity of speech and language therapy and provides guidance for ethically informed clinical decision making.

Realistic case studies written by a range of speech and language therapists from around the globe examine the decision-making process in speech and language therapy, providing a careful balance of clinical knowledge and expertise along with addressing the priorities and needs of the individual, and wider ethical considerations. Students and educators can debate real dilemmas faced by clinicians, taking diverse values and theoretical models into account to foster students' learning development.

This book is an invaluable resource for undergraduate and postgraduate students and lecturers in speech and language therapy programmes and clinical educators on placement. Charities working with children and adults with communication disorders may also benefit from this resource in training and assessments.

Maria Garraffa is an Associate Professor in Psycholinguistics at the University of East Anglia. Her research focuses on language disorders across the lifespan, decolonising language education and language development in children living in areas of conflicts.

Shin Ying Chu is an Associate Professor in Speech and Language Therapy at the National University of Malaysia. Her research focuses on speech motor control, particularly in disorders like Parkinson's disease and stuttering.

Neil Coull is a Lecturer in Speech and Language Therapy at the University of East Anglia and a qualified speech and language therapist. His clinical background involves working with adults with acquired communication, voice, and swallowing difficulties.

Julia Hubbard is an Emeritus Professor at the University of East Anglia with a clinical background in adult nursing. She is a highly experienced academic having worked in university level healthcare education since 1993 and has been involved in curriculum development and course delivery across a range of healthcare professions both nationally and internationally.

For more information about this series, please visit: https://www.routledge.com/Business-and-Decision-Making/book-series/[illegible]

Dilemmas and Decision Making

Series Editor: Julia Hubbard

Dilemmas and Decision Making in Social Work
Abbi Jackson

Dilemmas and Decision Making in Residential Childcare
Abbi Jackson

Dilemmas and Decision Making in Midwifery
A Practice-Based Approach
Edited by Kenda Crozier, Julia Hubbard

Dilemmas and Decision Making in Dementia Care
Sarah Housden, Julia Hubbard

Dilemmas and Decision Making in Policing
Emma Spooner, Bob Cooper

Dilemmas and Decision Making in Nursing
A Practice-Based Approach
Edited by Julia Hubbard

Dilemmas and Decision Making in Cancer Care
A Practice-Based Approach
Edited by Sarah Housden and Julia Hubbard

Dilemmas and Decision Making in Speech and Language Therapy
Edited by Maria Garraffa, Shin Ying Chu and Neil Coull

For more information about this series please visit https://www.routledge.com/Dilemmas-and-Decision-Making/book-series/CRITDADM

Dilemmas and Decision Making in Speech and Language Therapy

Edited by
Maria Garraffa, Shin Ying Chu, and Neil Coull

Series Editor: Julia Hubbard

Routledge
Taylor & Francis Group
LONDON AND NEW YORK

Designed cover image: Getty Images

First published 2026
by Routledge
4 Park Square, Milton Park, Abingdon, Oxon OX14 4RN

and by Routledge
605 Third Avenue, New York, NY 10158

Routledge is an imprint of the Taylor & Francis Group, an informa business

British Library Cataloguing-in-Publication Data
A catalogue record for this book is available from the British Library

ISBN: 978-1-041-13234-9 (hbk)
ISBN: 978-1-041-13227-1 (pbk)
ISBN: 978-1-003-66875-6 (ebk)

DOI: 10.4324/9781003668756

Typeset in Roboto
by Deanta Global Publishing Services, Chennai, India

Contents

About the editors

Maria Garraffa, PhD, FHEA, works as an Associate Professor in Speech and Language Sciences in the Faculty of Medicine and Health Sciences at the University of East Anglia (UEA). She does research on Communication Disorders Across the Lifespan, Decolonising Language Education and Bilingualism. Maria is passionate about supporting minority languages and language diversity in hard-to-reach communities. Internationally, she is Board member for the UK-Malaysia British Council, Honorary Fellow of Bilingualism Matters, and elected for the InterAcademy Partnership group (IAP) on Enhancing Global Scientific Exchange and Networking. She has authored several papers and books to inform policy makers on the effects of language learning and language revitalisation on individual and community well-being. She is currently an awardee for the Academy of Medical Sciences working on a research initiative in support of children living in areas of conflict.

Shin Ying Chu, PhD, is an Associate Professor in the Faculty of Health Sciences at the National University of Malaysia (UKM) and a certified speech and language therapist. She is passionate about advancing culturally responsive speech-language pathology practices across Asia and promoting evidence-based care for underserved communities. She has been awarded multiple competitive grants, including the Australia-APEC Women in Research Fellowship, APNIC Foundation's ISIF grant, Japan Society for the Promotion of Science (JSPS), and various national research funding schemes. She has authored numerous peer-reviewed publications and books addressing communication disorders, social participation outcomes, and cross-cultural therapeutic approaches. Currently, she leads international collaborations examining the social impact of communication disorders and developing AI-integrated healthcare solutions for allied health professionals across Southeast Asia.

Neil Coull is a qualified speech and language therapist and Lecturer in the Faculty of Medicine and Health Sciences at the University of East Anglia (UEA). His clinical background is in adult acquired speech and language therapy, working with individuals who have communication, voice, and swallowing difficulties. Neil has a clinical interest in voice disorders, dysphagia, and aphasia, and teaches in all those areas. In addition, Neil runs the Conversation Partners scheme which promotes social opportunities for people with aphasia through regular interactions with speech and language therapy students. Neil has contributed to peer-reviewed publications with an emphasis on promoting active client participation in therapeutic interactions.

Series editor:

Julia Hubbard is an Emeritus Professor of Clinical Health Education at the University of East Anglia (UEA) and a highly experienced academic having worked in university level healthcare education since 1993. During this time, she has been involved in curriculum review and development and course delivery across a range of healthcare professions at undergraduate and postgraduate levels, both nationally and internationally. Julia also holds honorary lectureships at the Royal Marsden School, London and Boromarajonani College of Nursing Chaing Mai, Thailand. Her current roles include series editor for the Dilemmas and Decision Making series and working as a QAA reviewer for Nursing and Midwifery Council approved curricula. In addition, she undertakes consultancy work with universities to assist in the development and review of their healthcare programmes, both nationally and internationally.

List of contributors

Lily Basley (University of East Anglia, UK) is a practising advanced speech and language therapist in paediatrics and Lecturer in Speech and Language Therapy. She has clinical interests in multilingualism, AAC, and additional needs, with a keen focus on practice education and the impact of clinical placements. She supports student placements through her NHS role and by facilitating the in-house community hub.

Martha-Louise Browell (University of East Anglia, UK) is a practising specialist speech and language therapist in adult learning disabilities and Lecturer at the University of East Anglia. Her clinical interests within learning disabilities practice include advanced communication skills, mental capacity, dysphagia, augmentative and alternative communication, positive behaviour support, and palliative and end-of-life care.

Jing Feng is a speech and language therapist and PhD candidate in Clinical Linguistics at the National University of Malaysia (UKM), and Linguistics Lecturer at Linyi University, China. She specialises in autism, social communication disorders, and family-centred interventions, with clinical work spanning Malaysia and China. She designs bilingual intervention strategies for autistic children and her non-literal Language Intervention Program in Shandong trains families and professionals in culturally tailored speech therapy.

Fernanda Dreux M. Fernandes (University of São Paulo, Brazil) is a Phonoaudiologist with Master's and PhD degrees, and has been a Professor on the Phonoaudiology programme at the University of São Paulo for 38 years. She has published over 120 papers, mentored over 40 graduate students, and served as President of the Brazilian Phonoaudiology Association. Currently Vice-President for Education of the International Association of Communication Sciences and Disorders (IALP), she has received numerous awards including SBFa's Merit Award and ASHA Fellowship.

Emma Ferris (University of East Anglia, UK) is an Associate Professor in Speech and Language Therapy at the University of East Anglia, working in higher education since 2015. Her clinical roles have spanned NHS settings including a regional Cleft Lip & Palate Team, complex needs, and educational settings. She is also founder and owner of an independent speech and language therapy team.

Veronica Fierro is an Assistant Professor at Delaware Valley University with research interests in assessment and treatment in bilingual populations, multiculturalism, and global issues in speech-language pathology. She holds Master's degrees in counseling psychology and speech-language pathology, plus a PhD in speech-language pathology from the University of Kansas. As a bilingual (English/Spanish) speech-language pathologist since 2001, she focuses on assessment and intervention in bilingual populations and multicultural issues.

Lauren Flannery (University of East Anglia, UK) is a specialist speech and language therapist and a Lecturer in the School of Health Sciences at the University of East Anglia. She teaches across pre- and post-registration programmes, focusing on developmental language delay and disorder, stammering, clinical practice, partnership working, and leadership. Qualified in 2006 with over 16 years of experience, she continues active clinical practice providing specialist services to children and young people with complex developmental communication disorders.

Nick Frizzel (Youth Justice Service Norfolk, UK) is a highly specialist speech and language therapist based in Norfolk. He qualified as a speech and language therapist in 2017 and has 8 years of experience in paediatric clinical practice across independent education, community NHS, and Youth Justice sectors.

Kirsty Harrison (University of East Anglia, UK) is an Associate Professor in Speech and Language Therapy at the University of East Anglia, working in higher education since 2008. She qualified as a speech and language therapist in 2002 and has served in clinical settings including acute, community, stroke rehabilitation and brain injury rehabilitation. She has co-authored book chapters and contributed to peer-reviewed journal articles about dysphagia and aphasia.

Elissa Manzi (University of East Anglia, UK) is a specialist speech and language therapist and Lecturer in Speech and Language Therapy at the University of East Anglia. She previously worked in adult settings including stroke rehabilitation with people with aphasia, dysarthria, dysphagia, and cognitive communication difficulties. She is a member of the British Aphasiology Society committee and recently established Norwich Aphasia Choir, supported by speech and language therapy students, with ongoing related research.

Mst. Mim Meherunnessa (University of Dhaka, Bangladesh) is a Lecturer in the Department of Communication Disorders at the University of Dhaka. She has clinical experience with clients with autism spectrum disorder, ADHD, Down syndrome, cerebral palsy, stuttering, and hearing disorders. She teaches stuttering, developmental learning disability, cleft lip and palate, and cognitive development, with primary research interests in identifying underlying language structure of individuals with communication disorders and fluency disorders.

Rachael Unicomb (University of Newcastle, Australia) is a Senior Lecturer for the Bachelor of Speech Pathology (Honours) programme at the University of Newcastle. Her teaching, research, and clinical interests centre around supporting individuals who stutter, with her 2015 PhD investigating treatment of co-occurring stuttering and speech sound disorders in young children. She continues stuttering research investigating treatment complexities, works with international collaborators, and maintains private practice supporting children, adolescents, and adults who stutter.

Introduction

Maria Garraffa

This book is primarily shaped from the viewpoint of health practitioners who provide essential support to individuals with speech, language, communication, and swallowing disorders. It contains real to life practical scenarios for examining clinical dilemmas and decisions, blending practical scenarios with theoretical frameworks. This approach allows you to reflect on your own values and beliefs, fostering a deeper understanding of ethical considerations in communication and swallowing disorder care. By relating personal practice to established models and contemporary concepts, you can enhance your professional expertise and support your ongoing development within the field.

Communication disorders, which include a broad spectrum of conditions such as aphasia, speech sound disorders, stuttering, voice disorders, and developmental language impairments, represent a critical aspect of the global health landscape. Globally, the prevalence of communication disorders has been increasing, with recent estimates suggesting that approximately 7.5% of the world's population experience some form of communication impairment (World Health Organization [WHO], 2021). This rise can be attributed to several factors, including greater awareness and diagnosis, as well as the proliferation of neurodegenerative diseases, traumatic brain injuries, and stroke incidents, which are common causes of acquired communication disorders. Furthermore, with aging populations worldwide, the incidence of age-related conditions such as dementia and aphasia is projected to expand, posing significant challenges for healthcare systems and practitioners alike (WHO, 2021).

Communication disorders are a major public health problem as they are a leading cause of social, educational, and occupational difficulties, affecting millions of individuals worldwide. The American Speech-Language-Hearing Association (ASHA, 2020) emphasises that early diagnosis and intervention are crucial in mitigating long-term consequences and improving outcomes for individuals with communication impairments. Furthermore, the Global Burden of Disease Study (Günther et al., 2020) highlights that communication disorders contribute substantially to

DOI: 10.4324/9781003668756-1

disability-adjusted life years (DALYs), underscoring their importance as a public health concern.

The future landscape of care for individuals with communication disorders faces numerous challenges, including ensuring equitable access to services, integrating innovative digital and assistive technologies, and providing holistic, person-centred approaches that respect individual preferences and cultural contexts. As communication is fundamental to human connection and participation, the complexity of these disorders requires practitioners to be adaptable, ethically aware, and informed by current evidence and theoretical advancements. This book is divided into three parts and aims to support professionals in navigating these challenges, fostering ethical decision-making, and promoting best practices that enhance the quality of life for individuals living with communication disorders.

Part 1: Giving patients a voice: sensitivity, integrity and empowerment

In this part, we explore the complexity of the Speech and Language Therapy (SLT) role working with individuals across the lifespan with a variety of health challenges associated with communication and swallowing difficulties. We look at the SLT role in giving patients a voice and empowering them to make their own decisions, as well as the associated ethical dilemmas. The scenarios examined here include how SLTs may pick up on the early signs of undiagnosed neurological conditions and the challenges of navigating this sensitively (David). Another considers the importance of the environment of those with language and communication disorders, as in the case of therapists in Youth services working in supporting a minor in the justice system (Clara) or in the context of a family closely supporting a young adult with severe learning disabilities (Paul). Sometimes the familiar environment can be challenging and the specific needs of people with a swallowing problem need to be carefully discussed with the individual to be effectively implemented and fully understood (Ibrahim).

Part 2: Working with significant others – family, friends and carers

The real success of Speech and Language Therapy comes from its application to the individual's real-life and surroundings. SLTs work not only with those who have communication and swallowing difficulties, but also their family members, carers, and friends. By doing so, therapists educate and advise others on how best to support the individual. This section explores the role of the SLT when working with those who have a key role to play in the individual's care or treatment, and often know the individual best. This is the norm in the case of bilingual clients with the involvement of an interpreter during the clinical sessions (Adrianna) to better integrate the family into the therapeutic targets by using their native language. Integrating therapeutic targets could be extremely challenging if there are risks factors around mental health in the family and complex family circumstances (Rosie). The whole family, including siblings, and parental career goals can be affected if not carefully considered, for example when planning intervention for a child with autism (Kevin). The integration of a young adult with communication disorders can be challenging also for the environment external to the family, where a lack of understanding of the individual's needs may lead to social isolation and ostracisation (Noah). Difficulties in integrating children with language and communication disorders in the educational setting are unfortunately not rare (Dale).

Part 3: Interdisciplinary working in speech and language therapy

Speech and Language Therapists work with individuals who often have complex medical, social and developmental needs. As such, the SLT role is but one of several professionals who work with and support individuals and their families. In this part, we explore the importance of the SLT working alongside other professionals and services. We explore complex scenarios where a careful balance is needed between independence and maintaining safety for an individual following a stroke, and how input from different healthcare professionals can support this (Samuel), or the effect that social isolation can have on the life of a person with aphasia (Bella). Post-traumatic disorders can be at the core of a speech disorder requiring a team of specialists and the family to work together (Diego).

How to use this book

Rather than a single, fixed pathway, this book invites you to choose how you engage with it. You might prefer to move through the case studies sequentially to build a structured understanding of communication disorders, or you can explore individual cases that speak directly to your current learning needs or clinical experience. Each case opens with a lifelike, though fictional, clinical scenario, sometimes told from the perspective of a Speech and Language Therapist, or other member of the multidisciplinary team. These scenarios are designed to bring you into the reality of speech and language practice, showing not just what professionals do but how they think, reason, and make decisions based on the evidence available at the time.

Throughout each case study, you will find highlighted notes in the margins that connect to relevant models, theories, and approaches. For SLTs, these might link to frameworks for swallowing assessment, evidence-based approaches to treating speech and language disorders, voice rehabilitation techniques, or principles of communication partner training. By exploring these concepts in the "further information" section at the end of each case, you can consolidate your theoretical knowledge and see how it applies to practical decision-making.

Reflections included at the end of the cases often illustrate the interdisciplinary role of the SLT, whose work flexibly spans prevention, assessment, intervention, and advocacy. Examples include working with patients to re-establish safe swallowing, introducing Augmentative and Alternative communication (AAC) when speech is compromised, or collaborating with oncologists to optimise communication outcomes.

At the end of each scenario, you will find a few reflective questions. These are designed to encourage critical thinking, not just about the case, but about your own clinical reasoning and learning. For SLT students, questions might prompt you to consider which assessment tools you would choose, how you would modify therapy for a patient with multiple conditions, or how you would explain your intervention plan to the wider multidisciplinary team.

Finally, each case study invites you to view the scenario through multiple angles, such as the needs of an older client, a multicultural family, a lack of resources, or a more complex disability. For SLTs, this is particularly relevant: cultural factors may shape a patient's willingness to engage with therapy, while psychosocial factors may affect adherence to rehabilitation exercises. Reflect on the features you naturally use and consider adding other dimensions to ensure your practice remains holistic, person-centred, and culturally sensitive.

References

American Speech-Language-Hearing Association (ASHA). (2020). ***Communicative disorders***. www.asha.org/policy/rp1993-00208/

Günther Deuschl, Ettore Beghi, Franz Fazekas, Timea Varga, Kalliopi A Christoforidi, Eveline Sipido, Claudio L Bassetti, Theo Vos, Valery L Feigin. (2020). The burden of neurological diseases in Europe: an analysis for the Global Burden of Disease Study 2017. ***Lancet Public Health***, 5: e551–67. DOI: 10.1016/S2468-2667(20)30190-0

World Health Organization (WHO). (2019). ***Disabilities and health: Programme and project information***.

World Health Organization (WHO). (2021). ***Global status report on the public health response to dementia***. www.who.int/publications/i/item/9789240033245.

Part 1

Giving patients a voice: sensitivity, integrity, and empowerment

Case study 1
David: what's in a voice?

Neil Coull

David's referral

I have been working as a Speech and Language Therapist (SLT) for around six months when I meet David. My role is to provide intervention for adults with acquired communication disorders. David was referred to my voice clinic from the Ear, Nose and Throat (ENT) department at his local hospital due to changes in his voice quality. He is a retired Caucasian gentleman in his late 60s with an unremarkable medical history. He lives with his wife, also retired, and they enjoy socialising with friends. David's main interest is lawn bowling, and he has represented his club nationally in bowling competitions.

Theory: Acquired communication disorders

Approach: SLT role

Approach: ENT investigation

Initial investigations

David is referred for an ENT diagnostic investigation after reporting concerns about a hoarse voice quality to his General Practitioner (GP). He is assessed using fibre-optic nasendoscopy. No concerning pathology is found and there is no obvious cause for his voice changes. He is referred on to voice therapy for further guidance on addressing his hoarse voice.

Approach: Referral process

Approach: Fibreoptic nasendoscopy assessment

Theory: Causes of voice difficulty

Theory: Voice

Patient interview

Soon after his ENT investigation, I meet David in my clinic and carry out a detailed case history.

Approach: Case history taking

'Hello David, my name's Neil and I am a Speech & Language Therapist. I understand you've been having some difficulties with your voice. Can you tell me a bit about them?'

'I have to admit, I was a surprised when the doctor suggested I come see you.' David replied.

'Surprised?' I say, *'Why was that?'*

DOI: 10.4324/9781003668756-3

'Well, I'm fine. I've just got a bit of a tickly throat. I don't need any therapy.' As he says this, he clears his throat. I notice too that as he speaks, his voice sounds hoarse.

'I guess I just want to find out what's been going on for you and see if there is anything I can suggest to help,' I respond, *'there can be lots of reasons why people's voices change or the throat feels tickly.'*

David looks down at the floor and replies softly: *'Like cancer.'*

I meet David's gaze: *'That can certainly be a cause but the ENT report suggested that wasn't a concern.'*

Value: Reassurance

'I was really worried about it' says David, *'you read so many horrible things'*.

'And what do you understand about your voice difficulties?' I ask.

'Well, the doctor at the throat department used a camera and had a look. That wasn't very pleasant – putting it up my nose, I mean. But he had a look in my voice box, and he said there was nothing there to worry about, but he wanted me to see you. I don't really understand why if everything's ok.'

Value: Consent

'Well, as I said, there are lots of reasons why people's voices change and I want to see if there is anything I can suggest that might help' I explain. *'Would it be ok if I asked you some questions so I can get a better idea of what might have caused your difficulties?'*

David nods in agreement.

Approach: Exploring cause and impact

I try to determine the nature of the voice difficulties by asking questions about when David first noticed them; whether they are constant or intermittent; whether they cause pain or discomfort and the impact they are having on him. I ask him if they are preventing him from doing the things he typically enjoys.

David replies: *'It was about two or three months ago, and I noticed I had this really rattly throat and a bit of a cough. My wife told me to see the doctor. I didn't want to bother him as it wasn't that bad. When it hadn't cleared up in a couple of weeks, I thought maybe I should get it checked out. That's when my doctor sent me to the throat clinic.'*

I continue my line of enquiry: *'And did you notice any changes to your voice at that time?'*

David paused for a moment before replying *'I suppose it must've changed – people kept asking me if I had a cold.'*

'And was it painful at all?'

'Only really when I was talking to my wife. She's a bit hard of hearing, you see, and I must speak quite loudly so she can hear me.'

'And has your voice changed at all since? Has it got any better or any worse?'

'I think I'm a little hoarser now, I suppose,' David says, *'but to be honest, it's not really causing me any problems. It was more just the worry of why it had changed. You know, if it was cancer.'*

As the consultation progresses, I ask David a series of questions relating to the symptoms and his lifestyle generally. This is to gain an impression of how he uses his voice in his everyday life and to determine whether any of his typical day-to-day activities might be causing his hoarseness. Alongside the case history, I listen carefully to David as he speaks, considering his voice quality, including the appropriateness of his vocal pitch and loudness and the pace of his speech. I observe his posture and his breath support when speaking. All of these can impact on how the voice sounds and how comfortable it is to speak, but none are particularly concerning here. My conclusion is that David is experiencing mild dysphonia. The probable cause is a combination of behavioural factors including poor hydration and having to speak loudly to his wife due to her hearing difficulties. It is also possible that he was raising his voice to an uncomfortable level over distance outdoors whilst bowling to speak with teammates. I give him some general voice care advice. For example, I

Theory: Dysphonia

Approach: Voice care

suggest that he turn down the volume on the TV or radio when conversing with others, so he does not have to speak over any background noise. I also encourage him to ensure his wife can see his face when speaking. David says he will try those things and be sure not to shout when bowling.

I suggest to David that we meet again in a month for a review to ensure the voice difficulty has not worsened. As David leaves the clinic, his case is relatively straight-forward. I anticipate discharging him from voice therapy after his follow-up review appointment.

Approach: Review

David's review

When David returns after a month, I am surprised to see several changes, not just in his voice but in the overall intelligibility of his speech. His hoarse voice has become more pronounced, his speech is slower and more laboured, and the individual sounds in his speech are less clearly articulated. Greater effort is needed to understand him now.

'How have things been since I last saw you?' I ask.

'I've been doing all the things you suggested,' David replies, *'but the thing is, everything feels like more of an effort. It feels like I am speaking with cottonwool in my mouth.'*

Despite recognising these changes myself, I do not want to cause him alarm, but nor do I want to ignore them.

Value: Sensitivity

'I can hear some changes in your speech,' I say, *'when did those begin?'*

David looked thoughtful, *'Over the last couple of weeks – my wife said she is finding it more difficult to understand me.'*

'And has anything else changed?'

'No, it just feels much more effortful to talk.'

Value: Professional role/ boundaries

The changes to his speech are particularly concerning to me as it is not typical for those with voice difficulties to experience such speech changes and therefore not what I anticipated seeing when he returns. However, I am mindful that it is not appropriate for the SLT to offer a medical diagnosis.

I tell David that I want to better understand why his speech has changed and that I would like to seek further guidance from my clinical supervisor. David agrees that I can record a sample of his speech to discuss with my clinical supervisor, and we plan to meet again the following week. I suggest that David continues to follow my advice from before and to contact me before we are due to meet again if he needs to.

Clinical supervision

Approach: Clinical supervision

I meet with my clinical supervisor, Rachael, soon after my review appointment with David.

I begin: *'I would like to discuss a case that seems a little unusual. One of my patients came into clinic for a routine review appointment, but he was very different to what I expected.'*

'How do you mean unusual?'

'Well, we first met about a month ago and he had some slight changes to his voice. His report from ENT was unremarkable, and it seemed as though he just needed some voice care advice and then a follow-up review.' I explain.

'And what happened at your review?'

'He seemed to be much worse. I mean, his voice quality had changed but so too had his speech intelligibility. That doesn't make sense to me, and I am worried it might not be a voice difficulty after all.'

'What do you think it might be?'

'I wonder if it might be something neurological. It's the changes to his speech that are puzzling me.'

'Can you explain what these changes are?'

'His speech was unclear. But when I met him a month ago, his speech was completely fine.'

I play the recording for my supervisor, pointing out the key features of his voice and speech that I am concerned about, namely that the changes in speech intelligibility are suggestive of dysarthria. We agree that David would benefit from a referral to neurology to investigate what might be causing the changes.

Theory: Dysarthria

Approach: Neurology

Referring on

I meet David for a review appointment the following week. His presentation is much as it was the week before. He continues to display signs of both a hoarse voice along with the same slow, laboured speech which is difficult to understand. I explain that, given the recent and unexplained changes to his speech, I want to refer him for a neurology consultation. David looks concerned and asks me what I think is wrong. I explain that I do not know but that a neurologist will be able to carry out investigations that will help to give answers. Without a clear diagnosis, it is difficult to provide further appropriate treatment at that time. We discuss some general strategies to protect his voice and to enable him to be understood by others, including writing down key words and using non-verbal communication alongside his speech.

David's diagnosis

David is seen by a neurologist soon after. After a series of tests, he receives a diagnosis of Motor Neurone Disease (MND). The early symptoms of MND can originate in the nerves controlling the motor movements for speech and voice production, as was the case for David. The diagnosis is of significant shock to David and his wife. It will cause significant changes to David's life including a gradual loss of his independence as the muscles controlling movement across his body begin to weaken. He soon requires support with most daily tasks, including personal care and assistance to mobilise.

Theory: MND

Next steps

David's diagnosis requires input from different health professionals. I continue to work with David, though in a different role now. I identify and introduce alternative approaches to communication as the muscles involved in speaking gradually lose strength and tone. In addition, I address difficulties with eating, drinking, and swallowing to ensure that David can gain sufficient nutrition and hydration whilst reducing the risk of him choking or aspirating. This is clearly a quite different approach from managing David's initial voice difficulties.

Approach: Multi-disciplinary team

Theory: Aspiration

Reflections

For a newly qualified therapist, I found this case challenging. I felt puzzled by the unexpected and sudden changes in his presentation between our first and second meeting. However, I was mindful not to cause him any distress. Clinical supervision helped me in making sense of a complex and unexpected presentation. It was appropriate to explain to David that I had concerns but not to offer any opinions on the possible cause, beyond it being potentially related to neurology. Whilst a referral to neurology was warranted, this had to be discussed sensitively with David.

Working with David subsequently made me realise the life-altering trajectory of progressive diseases. It also made me realise that it is not unusual for SLTs to spot the early signs of neurological disease. This is due to their unique understanding of the physical structures involved in human communication and in swallowing. SLTs often meet individuals who have experienced subtle changes in the processes governing communication and swallowing. However, this poses challenges, particularly to the novice therapist. Firstly, it would not be appropriate to offer our opinions on possible medical diagnoses to individuals. The diagnosing of neurological disease is complex and not simply based on observation of changes in speech and swallowing abilities. In addition, in many cases, our theories on the possible underlying cause may simply not be correct – something I have learned for myself in subsequent cases.

Questions for reflection and discussion

1. Why might patients seek advice for a hoarse voice?
2. What might it be like for individuals to receive news of a life-changing diagnosis?
3. What skills might be involved in working with individuals who receive distressing news?
4. What is the role of the SLT in supporting individuals who have received diagnoses?
5. What might it feel like for the SLT to work with people who have life-changing diagnoses?
6. Why is it important for SLTs to have supervision for complex cases?

Further reading

British Voice Association: https://britishvoiceassociation.org.uk/

Centre for Swallowing & Voice: www.ucdvoice.org/

MNDA (Motor Neuron Disease Association): www.mndassociation.org/

Orrell R W & Guiloff R J (2023). Clinical Aspects of Motor Neurone Disease. ***Medicine***. 51(9) 658–662

Further information

Theories

Acquired communication disorders relate to difficulties with speech, language, communication, or voice. These may develop suddenly or over time and are often, but not exclusively, due to neurological disease. The causes include stroke, traumatic brain injury, and progressive diseases, such as Parkinson's disease and Multiple Sclerosis.

Aspiration: food or fluids enter the lungs leading to a high risk of chest infection.

Causes of voice difficulty are multiple and often multi-faceted (Boone, 2014). In many cases, they are caused by the way in which individuals use their voices, often due to occupational need or related to hobbies and interests. However, they can also be caused by underlying pathologies (such as tumours); psychological or emotional causes; or by neurological disease (affecting the muscles controlling the various parts of the body involved in voice production, including the respiratory system and movement of the larynx itself).

Dysarthria is a difficulty with muscles involved in speaking, usually of a neurological cause (Duffy, 2019).

Dysphonia is a term used for the disordered voice. Its severity is dependent on the extent of changes in voice quality and the impact it is having on the individual (Mathieson, 2001).

Motor Neurone Disease (MND) is a progressive neurological disease. At the present time, there is no cure for MND, and the progression of the disease can be rapid. Individuals with MND gradually lose general physical movement, including the muscles involved in eating, drinking, and swallowing (Yorkston, 2013).

Voice is produced through the interplay of three key processes: respiration, phonation, and resonance. Respiration provides the power to our voices, enabling the vocal folds to vibrate rapidly. This vibration is called phonation, and in turn, it produces sound known as voicing. The sounds are then shaped by the spaces in the oral and nasal cavities, and articulators, including the tongue, to produce audible speech. This is known as resonance (Mathieson, 2001).

Approaches

Case history taking involves interviewing the individual to gain greater insight into the lived experience of their difficulties, including when they began and their impact. It is a key element when assessing voice disorders (Stemple et al., 2020).

Clinical supervision is an important part of an SLT's ongoing development providing a confidential space to discuss individual cases as well as to discuss the therapist's general development needs.

ENT investigation: in the UK, an examination by an ENT clinic is required for all patients reporting voice difficulties prior to being seen for voice therapy (Royal College of Speech & Language Therapists [RCSLT], 2019).

Exploring cause and impact: the causes of voice disorders are multi-factorial and addressing these as well as identifying the impact of the difficulties is part of the assessment process (Boone, 2014).

Fibreoptic nasendoscopy assessment: a camera is inserted through a nostril and fed through the nasal cavity to the pharynx (the throat) to visualise the larynx and vocal folds (Stemple et al., 2020). This is to rule out any structural changes to the larynx that might indicate an underlying disease, such as cancer (National Institute for Health and Care Excellence [NICE], 2025). The procedure is invasive but not painful.

Multi-disciplinary team: due to the complex nature of MND, individuals receive input and support from a wide multi-disciplinary team (MDT) including doctors, physiotherapists, occupational therapists, and specialist neurology nurses.

Neurology: neurologists are medical professionals who specialise in the functioning of the brain.

Referral process: it is common practice for all patients reporting changes in their voice quality to be screened by the ENT team in the first instance (RCSLT, 2019).

Review: follow-up review appointments enable therapists to monitor the success of their interventions, and to plan whether therapy should continue or cases be closed.

SLT role is to assess the impact of the communication impairment on the individual and, depending on the underlying causes, explore ways of improving elements of their communication through therapy, or to help them develop alternative or compensatory approaches to expressing themselves (RCSLT, 2019).

Voice care is an aspect of voice therapy designed to protect the voice from further damage. This is often by proposing changes to lifestyle or behaviour that are contributing to the difficulties (Ferrand, 2018).

Values

Consent: healthcare professionals should seek informed consent by explaining what they intend to do and seeking permission from individuals.

Professional role/boundaries: healthcare professionals should be aware of the scope of their practice. Stepping beyond this may cause harm or distress to individuals.

Reassurance: medical investigations can be troubling and frightening for individuals. Healthcare professionals should address anxieties and concerns appropriately.

Sensitivity: healthcare professionals must be honest but should also consider how they discuss potentially distressing news with individuals.

References

Boone D (2014). The Voice and Voice Therapy. Pearson.

Duffy J R (2019). Motor Speech Disorders: Substrates, differential diagnosis, and management (4th ed.). Elsevier.

Ferrand C T (2018). Speech Science: An integrated approach to theory and clinical practice (4th ed.). Pearson.

Mathieson L (2001). The Voice & its Disorders (6th ed.). Whurr.

National Institute for Health and Care Excellence (NICE) (2025). Head and Neck Cancers – Recognition and Referrals. https://cks.nice.org.uk/topics/head-neck-cancers-recognition-referral/diagnosis/symptoms-suggestive-of-head-neck-cancers/

Royal College of Speech & Language Therapists (RCSLT) (2019). Voice – Guidance. www.rcslt.org/members/clinical-guidance/voice/voice-guidance/

Stemple J C, Roy N & Klaben B (2020). Clinical Voice Pathology: Theory and management (6th ed.). Plural.

Yorkston KM (2013). Management of Speech and Swallowing Disorders in Degenerative Diseases. Pro-Ed.

Case study 2
Paul: does he need this?

Martha-Louise Browell

Meeting Paul and his parents

I meet Paul for the first time at the home he shares with his parents. They are also present throughout the visit. I introduce myself, the purpose of the session and seek consent to undertake an assessment of his eating, drinking and swallowing. Having awareness of his communicative abilities, I adapt my communication by prioritising eye contact, tone of voice and body language to connect with Paul. I note that he has difficulties understanding and using language and this is consistent with his diagnosis of profound and multiple learning disabilities (PMLDs). For example, his expression consists of subtle changes in facial expression and tone of vocalisations; he does not use any forms of symbolic communication such as speech, signs or picture-symbols and his comprehension presents at a 'situational' level, meaning he can apprehend familiar cues, but has limited understanding of language, particularly relating to concepts outside of the here and now. I therefore have reason to question his capacity. I assess his understanding regarding the decision in question: whether to consent or refuse to have an assessment of dysphagia, and subsequently to make decisions around dysphagia management. I ask him to follow simple instructions and respond to basic questions using vocabulary relevant to the decision and accompanying these with non-verbal cues. For example, I ask *'Paul, show me your tongue'* and *'Paul, where is your tummy?'*. Questions such as these allow me to explore Paul's comprehension of basic vocabulary related to body structures involved in eating, drinking and swallowing. I triangulate my observations of his responses with my clinical impression of his communication skills across the appointment. From this, I conclude that Paul cannot understand the information via any means. I deem him to lack capacity to consent to the assessment as he cannot understand the basic information related to eating and drinking. It is reasonable to

Approach: Consent

Theory: PMLDs

Approach: Assessing capacity

Theory: Dysphagia

DOI: 10.4324/9781003668756-4

conclude he is unable to understand more complex information such as risks associated with dysphagia.

Paul's parents do not have legal authority to make decisions on his behalf, so the appointment continues in his best interests in order to ensure he is able to eat and drink as safely as possible. Paul and his parents engage willingly. I observe Paul throughout the appointment to make sure he is content and is participating voluntarily.

Approach: Best interests

Gathering information

I gather a case history from Paul's parents as I am unable to get the information directly from him. Prior to the appointment I had reviewed the referral information and patient summary from his GP. However, during the appointment I gather more detailed information about Paul's day-to-day experiences. I use an open question to gain his parents' perspectives, asking, '*Could you tell me about your thoughts and observations of Paul's eating & drinking?*'

Approach: Case history taking

'*All seems fine really*', they respond.

I try to encourage some elaboration from them, saying, '*Perhaps you could you describe how you support Paul to eat and drink, so I can get a bit of a picture.*'

'*Well, we obviously sort the food out for him. I give him small pieces at a time, and he can't hold a cup, so I give him his drinks with a straw*', Paul's mum responds.

'*Thank you and do you notice any coughing when he eats or drinks?*' I ask.

'*Erm, I don't think so....no, not really,*' replies his mum.

'*How about any chest infections? Has he had any over the last 6 months or so?*', I ask, to gather specific clinical information.

His mum thinks for a moment, '*No. He doesn't really get them.*'

'That's helpful to know,' I say, *'Thank you. So, the referral did mention that his respite team have worries over Paul coughing when he eats and drinks. They think he has had a chest infection too, although it is possible that was a seasonal infection. It would be helpful for me to observe Paul eating and drinking to see if there are any signs of difficulty. Or maybe there are things you are doing naturally to support him which I can share with his respite team. Would that be OK with you?'*

'Yes, alright,' says his mum.

It becomes clear that Paul's parents do not think he has any difficulties with EDS (eating, drinking and swallowing). However, the referral and GP's summary indicate otherwise, suggesting that an assessment is needed. Paul's parents are accepting of me continuing. Although the assessment is in Paul's best interests, I pay close attention to his demeanour throughout, so I can monitor his reactions to ensure he is not in distress.

Theory: EDS

Clinical swallow examination

Next, I observe Paul eating and drinking. Paul's mum prepares cheese on crackers and a drink. These equate to Level 7 'regular diet' and Level 0 'thin fluids' in the International Dysphagia Diet Standardisation Initiative (IDDSI) framework. Paul is supported to eat and drink as he does not have the fine motor skills to handle crockery and cutlery for himself. He eats in his specialist wheelchair which provides adequate postural support.

Theory: IDDSI framework

Theory: Postural stability

I look and listen for cues to assess different aspects of Paul's swallow. He cannot tolerate hands-on assessment methods, such as palpation and auscultation. Therefore, I visually observe the movement of his oral musculature, the efficiency of mastication (chewing) and how well he can form the food into a cohesive shape/size (or bolus) for swallowing. I look and listen for signs of penetration-aspiration, including monitoring the range of movement in his larynx.

Theory: Stages of swallow

Approach: Palpation

Approach: Auscultation

Theory: Penetration-aspiration

I notice Paul has very limited jaw and tongue motion meaning the food was not prepared/organised into a cohesive bolus that is easy to swallow. Food residue is present across his mouth, which increases the potential risk of food particles going into the airway. Paul coughs with visible facial flushing and eye-tearing when offered a drink, using a straw. The severity of the coughing suggests this has been a deep penetration or aspiration.

Initial findings

I feedback my initial observations to Paul's parents. They wonder if this presentation is because of issues with his seating, which is relevant to question due to his severe scoliosis. However, I reassure them his seating position is appropriate; allowing his mouth and larynx to be in alignment and providing proximal postural stability. I share my hypothesis that Paul is unable to form a cohesive bolus, leaving residue in his mouth, and that using a straw creates rapid flow which he is unable to control, resulting in fluid and residue moving rapidly into his airway.

Exploring the hypothesis

I ask to see Paul eat a banana, which is considered an example of IDDSI level 6: 'soft & bite-sized' foods. Paul is given small pieces of it. He effectively chews and prepares this with significantly less residue. His tongue and jaw movements are sufficient to manage this texture. I ask his mum to wait until his mouth is clear before offering him anything to drink, to reduce the chance of penetration-aspiration. Paul is then supported to take small sips of water from a regular cup. He manages without any coughing, flushing or tearing. Sipping from a cup offers him more control than sucking on a straw.

Feeding back findings

After the observation I explain the core aspects of EDS to Paul's parents, *'For us to chew and swallow well we need to use our jaw and tongue to make the food soft and collected in the mouth so we can swallow this easily. There are lots of muscles and structures involved to make sure the top of the airway is covered when we swallow and that food or drink goes where it is meant to go – down the oesophagus towards the stomach. Does that make sense?'*

Paul's parents nod and smile.

I continue, '*What's happening for Paul is that he has less movement in his jaw and tongue, meaning food isn't formed into a nice easy shape for swallowing. Instead, particles are splitting and spreading across his mouth, which makes it much trickier for him to swallow these without pieces going into his airway. When drinking through a straw, the fluid is rushing towards the back of the mouth before the airway is safely covered. The risk is that this increases his chance of food or drinks going down to his lungs and causing infections.*'

I pause to allow time for comments and to gauge whether Paul's parents are following.

'*Any questions so far?*' I ask.

'*No, that's fine*', Paul's mum replies.

'*Ok. Please do say if you'd like me to repeat anything or go over anything again*', I say, '*In terms of what we do next, there are three approaches that I would recommend. These are on top of what you are already doing well around making sure Paul is sitting well in his chair and supporting him to eat/drink. First, use a cup instead of a straw. Second, give a small gap between foods and fluids so that his mouth is clear. And third is to move to what's called 'IDDSI 6 soft and bite-sized'. This is a way of describing different textures of foods, to help us be consistent and clear with what we offer someone.*' I share a leaflet about IDDSI 6 with them, including the testing methods, highlighting the size and texture requirements.

Value: Accessible information

I continue, '*For Paul, this helps with removing some of the more difficult textures and gives him a head-start, if you like, with chewing. Many foods can be cooked or prepared in a way that makes them IDDSI 6. Can you talk me through what Paul's favourite foods are and what he tends to eat at each meal?*' I ask this to ensure that Paul is not unduly restricted with his eating.

Value: Ethics and eating

We identify that Paul likes a wide range of foods, without any particular preferences. Other than crumbly or chewy foods, such as crackers and crackling, all the other foods he typically enjoys could be easily prepared as IDDSI 6.

Reflections

There were three aspects of this situation that made this case challenging. The first of these is the challenge of clinical decision making when an individual is unable to advocate for themselves. The second is related to this and involves establishing effective communication and rapport with family members who support the individual's care. The third dilemma relates to the research evidence base to support individuals with PMLDs with their swallowing difficulties.

Decision making when the person is unable to advocate for themselves

I felt relaxed and confident in my interactions with Paul, using non-verbal communication such as eye contact to develop rapport. I felt sure of my impression he lacked capacity to consent. I observed his non-verbal presentation throughout the appointment and noted he appeared content, engaging in play with his favourite objects. This reassured me that continuing with the appointment was OK for him.

Supporting decision-making capacity is a legal obligation under the Mental Capacity Act (Parliament of the United Kingdom, 2005). I was prepared to support communication with Paul to maximise his autonomy and ability to consent. As an experienced Speech and Language Therapist (SLT) in the field of Adult Learning Disabilities (ALD) I used intuitive reasoning processes to identify patterns in his non-verbal communication, e.g., the way he responded to me, those familiar to him and his environment. I formed an impression of his communication which supported my assessment and reasoning around his capacity as well as helping me to feel confident that my presence and the process of assessment was not causing distress.

Rapport and interaction with significant others

In contrast to how I felt communicating with Paul, I felt self-conscious with his parents. I was aware from Paul's electronic record that his dad could be abrupt and dismissive with professionals. Neither of his parents were overtly warm and welcoming on arrival, e.g., there was limited eye contact and social greetings. I felt they were evaluating me, causing me to feel greatly aware of what I was saying and how. Listening to their criticisms of other healthcare professionals made me feel uneasy, concerned they may feel similarly towards me and that this would impede a successful outcome for Paul.

However, it was vital I worked to communicate well with them to ensure I was in accordance with legal and professional guidance by involving them in assessment and decision making. Although they did not have legal grounds to consent or refuse on his behalf, they had valuable insight and were integral to supporting him.

I remained calm and attentive throughout, listening and responding to what they said. I avoided colluding in their criticisms of other professionals, opting instead to empathise with their perceptions and suggesting ways we could progress with the issues.

I was mindful to balance encouraging them to share their full perspective, whilst also ensuring I gathered the information needed about Paul's EDS. I was aware their primary concern regarding positioning may be acting as a barrier to them noticing EDS dysfunction. A technique used to do this was through specific question types. Open questions enabled Paul's parents to speak freely about his experiences, whilst closed questions were helpful in gaining specific, targeted information about his EDS.

During the discussion I felt Paul's mum was attentive and engaged, whereas I perceived Paul's dad as being more reticent. He remained standing during the conversation and did not come over to look at the resources. His comments were typically short with a firm tone. I tried to mitigate this by being open and collaborative. I utilised clinical communication skills, as one of four essential aspects for clinical competence (Kurtz, Silverman and Draper, 2005) along with knowledge, problem solving and examination skills. I used techniques such as social commenting, eye contact and body posture to present as relaxed and attentive as well as using a range of question types. I also had resources ready to discuss management strategies, however I realised that it would also have been useful to have diagrams/models ready to explain the process of EDS.

Decision making in the context of a limited research evidence base

The evidence base for management of dysphagia in the field of ALD is sparse, despite high prevalence of the condition. In a well-reported systemic review, Manduchi, Fainman and Walshe (2020) identified only four articles addressing management of dysphagia in ALD. All discussed enteral feeding only and had limited methodological rigour. Consequently, assessment and management are a highly intuitive process, consisting of active problem solving and characterised by reasoning across the first three modes of Standing's Cognitive Continuum: intuitive judgement, reflective judgement and patient-aided judgement (Standing, 2010).

The Lens Model (Standing, 2010) proposes that during the process of assessment the clinician gathers 'cues' to understand the situation and inform decisions. The utility and validity of these cues need to be considered to enable an accurate judgement. Having reviewed Paul's record, I was aware his parents tended to have reservations about working with professionals and could be guarded in their manner. This knowledge informed my assessment of cue validity and utility; for example, listening attentively to their descriptions and concerns around positioning, recognising that this is relevant to dysphagia management but not disregarding the possibility of further contributing factors. I could have taken their reports of an absence of EDS difficulties at face-value and concluded there was no indication to proceed. However, I chose not to take this approach as I was aware that his parents may decline assessment prematurely. By gathering information with consideration of validity and utility, I was able to prepare for direct EDS observation with an open mind, i.e., minimising the risk of anchoring bias, where the clinician attaches to an early interpretation and fails to refine hypotheses when new evidence is revealed (Cooper and Frain, 2016).

During the observation I felt confident I had witnessed penetration-aspiration. I felt concerned for Paul and surprised he had not been experiencing aspiration pneumonias. However, it was possible he had a high tolerance to aspiration, as aspiration alone does not always result in pneumonia (Nativ-Zeltzer et al., 2021).

I thought Paul's mum appeared shocked by what she had seen, due to changes in her facial expression and her engagement with me. Paul's dad seemed less concerned; however, his affect is quite different and he wasn't as close at the time.

After the assessment I talked through my findings and recommended strategies, gaining their insight and knowledge of Paul and his preferences to guide the decision making. I noticed myself feeling confident with this and remembered a time when I was training that I would not have felt so clear. I explained what aspiration was and why this was a risk, however I could have linked this more to what Paul may be experiencing, e.g., discomfort and distress. This may have been more impactful for them, given their care for Paul.

When discussing texture modification as one form of managing Paul's dysphagia, I found that a lot of the foods we discussed appeared to be suitable for IDDSI 6 recommendations. However, I was concerned that they may have been selectively describing how they prepare food, so they were following this level already. There is no way to know how accurate their reports are without intruding on their home life, but I attempted to explore their narrative and discuss as many examples as possible.

During the conversation I looked for signs of understanding from Paul's parents, i.e., through their engagement and relevance of comments. I could have more actively checked what they were taking from the conversations and on reflection I do not feel confident they will implement the strategies we agreed.

Decisions for Paul were guided by flexibly applying knowledge to his presentation. For example, I observed Paul to have oral and pharyngeal stage dysfunction so problem solving was used to trial alternatives in equipment, texture and support technique. Fortunately, these mitigated the apparent dysfunction; however, should these have been ineffective, further trials would have been conducted. I discussed the impact of these strategies specifically for Paul, balancing my clinical knowledge of risk/safety with their knowledge of him and how he eats/drinks on a day-to-day basis. This combined approach allowed us to develop an initial management plan for him.

Questions for reflection and discussion

1. What thoughts and feelings are generated for you following reading this case study?
2. What would you try to do similarly when interacting with the individual and their family members and why?
3. What would you try to do differently and why?
4. How do you think you would feel trying to understand and meet the needs of someone who cannot advocate for themselves?
5. What materials/resources or approaches could you use to support communication with Paul and with his parents?
6. What else do you think SLT could do for Paul, following this appointment?

Further reading

Jones, I. and Volkmer, A. (Eds) (2019). ***Speech and Language Therapists and Mental Capacity*: *A training resource for adult services.*** J & R Press.

Marks, L. and Rainbow, D. (2001). ***Working with Dysphagia***. Speechmark.

Nicholson, C., Finlay, W. M. L. and Stagg, S. (2023). Self-determination and co-operation in supported mealtimes involving people with severe intellectual disabilities. ***Disability and Rehabilitation 45*** (17), 2741–2750.

Robertson, J., Chadwick, D., Baines, S., Emerson, E. and Hatton, C. (2018). People with intellectual disabilities and dysphagia. ***Disability & Rehabilitation 40*** (11), 1345–1360.

Royal College of Speech and Language Therapists. (2023). ***Position Paper: Learning Disabilities (children, young people and adults).*** RCSLT. www.rcslt.org/wp-content/uploads/2023/03/RCSLT-Learning-Disabilities-position-paper-2023.pdf

Further information

Theories

Dysphagia is a medical term relating to difficulties swallowing (Logemann, 1998).

EDS (eating, drinking and swallowing) is increasingly used by Speech and Language Therapists (SLTs) in place of the more medicalised term, dysphagia, to be more inclusive of the wider range of factors influencing how an individual meets their nutrition and hydration needs.

IDDSI framework is used to describe texture/consistency modification for dysphagia. Alterations to texture/consistency is one approach to dysphagia management (Cichero et al., 2017).

Penetration-aspiration: these terms relate to food and fluid entering the airway rather than the oesophagus. Penetration refers to when food/fluid enters the upper larynx whereas aspiration refers to food/fluid going deep into the larynx and/or into the airway and lungs. Instrumental assessment is needed to fully assess extent of penetration-aspiration; however, clinical signs such as change in voice quality, coughing and facial flushing can suggest that penetration-aspiration has occurred (Logemann, 1998).

Postural stability is needed to underpin stability and functioning of the oropharyngeal musculature involved in eating/drinking/swallowing.

PMLDs (profound and multiple learning disabilities). This is where a person has a severe-profound level of intellectual disability along with other physical/sensory conditions.

Stages of swallow: the oral stage primarily involves mastication of food and preparation of food/fluid into a safe bolus for transitioning to the oropharynx. The pharyngeal stage refers to the passage of the bolus over the airway into the oesophagus, ensuring the airway is protected (Logemann, 1998).

Approaches

Assessing capacity: where mental capacity regarding a specific decision is questioned, it needs to be established whether the person can understand, retain and weigh-up the relevant information and then communicate their decision. Inability in one of these areas, despite maximum support being provided, means the person lacks capacity at that time for that decision. Capacity is time and decision specific, so a person may have capacity to make some decisions and not others (Parliament of the United Kingdom, 2005).

Auscultation: listening to sounds during swallowing, e.g., breath sounds immediately before and after the swallow (Cichero and Murdoch, 2006).

Best interests: this is a decision-making process when the individual does not have the capacity to make the decision. All relevant people should be involved (such as the person's family/care team, relevant professionals and sometimes a professional advocate) and able to discuss all available options together. The person who will be enacting the outcome of the decision is usually the 'decision-maker', e.g., a GP prescribing a medication, a surgeon operating on the person or a therapist providing assessment/therapy. The degree of formality can vary depending on the complexity of the decision, the impact of the possible outcomes and the degree of agreement/discord amongst those involved. The person's own views and feelings should be incorporated to the greatest extent possible.

Case history taking is a critical part of assessment, underpinning hypotheses and management plans.

Consent consists of three aspects: it must be informed, voluntary and capacitous. This is a core legal and professional requirement when providing healthcare. Everyone should be assumed to be able to make a capacitous decision, unless there is indication otherwise and they have 'an impairment of their mind or brain' which could influence capacity (Parliament of the United Kingdom, 2005).

Palpation: feeling the coordination and range of movement in the base of the tongue and laryngeal structures (Logemann, 1998).

Values

Accessible information: healthcare professionals have a duty to present information in a way which is understandable for the audience regardless of their knowledge or literacy. It is good practice when providing a leaflet to discuss this with the person and highlight/explore areas which are particularly relevant to their situation.

Ethics and eating: management of dysphagia is multi-factorial and not only around reducing aspiration risk. Any recommendations made by Speech and Language Therapists should not be unduly restrictive in terms of what individuals can eat, nor should they impact on quality of life.

References

Cichero, J.A.Y., Lam, P., Steele, C.M., Hanson, B., Chen, J., Dantas, R.O., Duivestein, J., Kayashita, J., Lecko, C., Murray, J., Pillay, M., Riquelme, L. and Stanschus, S. (2017). Development of international terminology and definitions for texture-modified foods and thickened fluids used in dysphagia management: the IDDSI Framework. ***Dysphagia 32***, 293–314.

Cichero, J.A.Y. and Murdoch, B.E. (Eds.) (2006). ***Dysphagia: Foundation, Theory and Practice.*** Wiley & Sons.

Cooper, N. and Frain, J. (2016). ***ABC of Clinical Reasoning.*** Wiley-Blackwell.

Kurtz, S., Silverman, J. and Draper, J. (2005). ***Teaching and Learning Communication Skills in Medicine*** (2nd ed.). Radcliffe Publishing.

Logemann, J.A. (1998). ***Evaluation and Treatment of Swallowing Disorders*** (2nd ed). Pro-ed.

Manduchi, B., Fainman, G.M. and Walshe, M. (2020). Interventions for feeding and swallowing disorders in adults with intellectual disability: a systematic review of the evidence. ***Dysphagia 35***, 207–219.

Nativ-Zeltzer, N., Nachalon, Y., Kaufman, M.W., Seeni, I.C., Bastea, S., Aulakh, S.S., Makkiyah, S., Wilson, M.D., Evangelista, L., Kuhn, M.A., Sahin, M. and Belafsky, P.C. (2021). Predictors of aspiration pneumonia and mortality in patients with dysphagia. ***Laryngoscope 132***, 1172–1176.

Parliament of the United Kingdom (2005). ***Mental Capacity Act.*** www.legislation.gov.uk/ukpga/2005/9/contents

Standing, M. (Ed.) (2010). ***Clinical Judgement and Decision-Making in Nursing and Interprofessional Healthcare*** (pp. 108–128). McGraw-Hill Education.

Case study 3
Clara: finding a voice in the Youth Justice System

Nick Frizzell

Background and referral

Clara is a 16-year-old girl who is looked after by the Local Authority (LA). She previously lived with her father, who is separated from Clara's biological mother. Her mother is reported to have had substance misuse issues throughout Clara's life. Clara has been referred to the Youth Justice Service (YJS) by the Police and court due to several criminal offences. She has been referred to the Youth Justice Speech and Language Therapy (SLT) team following concerns around her engagement and understanding. Following an increase in the frequency of offences, including possession of Class B drugs, Clara has been given a referral order for twelve months and given a Global Positioning System (GPS) tag to ensure she does not enter an exclusion zone put in place by the court. She likes to play football but does not really follow a team. Other interests tend to come and go, depending on her mood, and she says that she is bored most of the time and just wants '*to go out with mates.*'

I book an appointment to see her at her home to build up a picture of how she communicates. Before meeting her, I call her dad to gather some background information. I ask him how Clara has been getting on at school.

Approach: Case history taking

'*She's always struggled at school*', he says, '*when she was in Primary, the teachers said she was always hiding under the table.*'

'*Did she have any favourite subject?*' I ask.

'*No, she's not one for books*', he thinks for a moment, '*To be fair, I wasn't a great fan of school either – I was always much better with my hands.*'

DOI: 10.4324/9781003668756-5

'And how are things with Clara at school at the moment?' I ask him.

'She doesn't go at the moment – she hasn't been going for a while now', he says, going on to explain that Clara has experienced multiple fixed term and permanent exclusions from school including specialist provision for Social, Emotional and Mental Health (SEMH).

'What do you think she is finding hard about school?' I ask him.

'I really couldn't tell you' he says, *'there was talk at one point about dyslexia or something, I'm not too sure. I don't think that ever went anywhere'*. He pauses, *'She's really restless, you see – always has been. Her teachers never knew what to do with her'*.

I thank Clara's dad for his time. It has been helpful to get some background information from someone who knows her well.

Theory: Dyslexia

I then check her case notes and record. It says she has never been formally assessed for dyslexia as she has not been able to tolerate a full assessment. Her record shows she does not have contact with her biological mother, apart from chance meetings in the local area. Clara told her YJS case manager that she recently saw her mum and went to hug her, but her mum did not hug her back. Professionals have noted a deterioration in Clara's mental health following these brief interactions and she has made two attempts on her life in the last year. She has also been frequently arrested for drunken and disorderly behaviour prior to appearances in court.

Assessing Clara

I arrange to meet Clara at her placement – a Local Authority *Supports Living* home with live-in support staff – with a familiar and trusted Youth Justice Mental Health practitioner. It was expected that Clara would be anxious around a new professional and that her engagement may suffer if she were expected to meet with me alone.

Within community paediatric speech and language teams, it is typical practice to use standardised assessment tools to gather evidence of any presenting Speech, Language and Communication Needs (SLCN), however, with knowledge of Clara's education background and engagement, it was deemed that an approach using dynamic assessment would be more appropriate.

Theory: SLCN

Approach: Dynamic assessment

A visual scale from the Language for Behaviour and Emotions (LfBE) resource is used to gain Clara's own views of her communication. Clara places the majority under *'tricky sometimes,'* however, initial responses are sometimes *'don't know'* and occasionally she asks, *'what does that mean?'* She places narrative skills (*'How easy or tricky is it to tell someone who wasn't there all the details about something that happened?'*) under *'easy.'*

Approach: LfBE

An informal assessment is conducted looking at her ability to remember and understand information, recall spoken sentences and emotional vocabulary, and use her narrative skills. Observations of her form and content of her language, word finding and social communication are made through conversation with her.

Assessment of Clara's communication is carried out using subtests of the CELF-5 (see Wiig, Semel and Secord, 2013). Clara presents with difficulties in all areas of communication that are assessed, particularly with verbal memory and narrative skills. Her recall of spoken sentences is significantly limited with half of the sentences (7/14) containing errors which change the meaning of the message. This includes forgetting words and parts of sentences and changes to words. For example, Clara is asked to repeat the target sentence: *'The class who sells the most tickets to the dance will win a prize.'* She says: *'The class that wins the most tickets will win a prize.'*

Approach: CELF-5

A narrative assessment from the LfBE is used, where the child is asked to listen to a story and then retell it in their own words. Clara is able to recall minimal information, omitting characters, key events, internal responses, plans, actions of the character and a conclusion. An example of her retelling of one of the stories is as follows: *'The person went to their mates' house and um like for food and at school they got told off. And I forgot.'* A child without speech and language needs would typically be able to give a simple, but complete, story, and the listener would be able to build a picture in their own mind of what happened and why it was important. Clara's story here is incomplete, lacking salient details from the source material.

Approach: Assessing emotion

Clara is asked to match a set of given scenarios relating to emotional state. For example, she is asked how someone might feel attending a job interview; she is unable to give a response, saying, *'I don't know how to explain it.'* When given the scenario of a child falling over in a race and hearing people laugh at them, she responds only when given forced alternatives of *'embarrassed'* or *'frustrated.'* She points to *'embarrassed.'* This test reveals the difficulties she has in expressing emotions.

Clara engages in a full assessment session of just under one hour, frequently looking at her phone for up to 30 seconds at a time before responding or requesting the question to be repeated. The mental health practitioner present comments that this is typical for Clara. It seems that this is a strategy Clara uses to allow herself processing time and to mask her communication difficulties.

Clara's assessment results show difficulties with receptive and expressive language and other higher level language skills such as reasoning, negotiating, problem solving and inferencing, all of which are impacting her engagement in daily life. These difficulties are reported to have been persistent and consistent with a diagnosis of DLD (Developmental Language Disorder). However, given her early developmental trauma and education history, it is difficult to determine whether she presents with a specific disorder or whether she has simply not had the opportunity to learn and develop language at a young age. This makes diagnosing Clara more challenging.

Theory: Narrative competence

From what I have seen firsthand and from others' accounts, Clara can appear to be uncaring of the thoughts, feelings and beliefs of others and does not appear to learn from her mistakes. From her assessment, I hypothesise that she is, in fact, unable to generate a complete narrative about events in her life with her own perspective and that of others.

After assessing Clara, I share my findings and hypotheses about how Clara's SLCN might be impacting her daily life with others, including her Social Worker, Youth Justice Officer, Placement staff and her dad. Clara's dad says how much it all makes sense and *'no wonder she couldn't do school.'* I record my findings in a report written for Clara following a Child-First approach as well as a communication profile. Shortly after her assessment is completed, Clara is moved from supported living to a semi-independent placement, where the level of adult support is reduced significantly overnight. She is moved due to other children needing a place rather than her being deemed ready to move.

Approach: Child-First

Actions and consequences

During a follow up visit to her new placement, I speak with Clara about her experiences of court and her misuse of cannabis the night before her football club match:

'How do you find it when you are in court?' I ask

Clara responds, *'It's like they're speaking a different language.'*

'That must be hard,' I say, *'I would feel confused and frustrated if I did not know what was happening to me.'*

Clara looks despondent, *'I don't care; I just don't listen.'*

'And how's football going?' I ask.

'Alright,' she says.

'I heard you were smoking again,' I say, *'What do you think your coach would say if he knew you were smoking weed before matches?'*

Clara shrugs, *'How would I know?'*

'Well, if I was the coach I might think...' I begin, before pausing momentarily.

Clara quickly interjects, *'How would you know what they think?'*

Theory: Theory of mind

Although impossible to say for certain, the tone with which she says this seems more curious in nature than intolerant of the conversation. Through further exploration of Clara's mentalising, narrative and inferencing skills, she continues to present as not yet being able to conceptualise and understand the inner mental states of others. Considering Clara's early development and parental behaviour and upbringing (from the limited background history information available), I hypothesise that her parents may not have been able to help her develop her own theory of mind. In Clara's notes, one report from placement staff refers to her dad's own poor mentalisation when he undermined staff's authority in front of Clara, *'If she wants to do it, just let her.'* He possibly does not understand the impact that his words and actions have had on her respecting the boundaries and rules in place to safeguard her. That night, she ignores staff as they advise her not to go out, saying *'It's fine, my dad doesn't care.'* She stays out until 2am, drinking alcohol. She calls staff to come pick her up and vomits out the car window on the way back home.

Clara tells me stories, not through oral narratives, but her social media stories. She says 'look' and holds her smart phone out for me to see her with friends out in the community. Her connectives within stories are marked by *'see this, yea'* and *'and then we went here, yea, and then we just did nuffin, yea, but the police just got Noah and we all legged it,'* with description of the actions of her and others, but rarely reference to the inner mental states of the story's characters. She also often omits a resolution to the stories, and no evaluation of the significance of the event and the impact on others. An example of this is when she describes claiming food from the collection point at a popular fast-food restaurant belonging to another customer. In her recounting, she does not attempt to express any thought towards the individual whose order she had stolen. Rather, her account is limited to wanting to eat and taking the food. When I press her, she is unable to say what the consequence might be if she were to return to the same location. Many of Clara's arrests are reported to be the result of being unable to give a positive account of herself when under suspicion from reporting officers. This has led to physical manifestations of her frustrations including the assault of an emergency worker when being detained.

Theory: Narrative skills

Supporting Clara

In meetings with the professional network and within Clara's communication profile, I share my hypothesis that her difficulty with narrative likely impacts and impairs her ability to construct internal monologues. I raise the consideration that existing expectations for her to independently think about, reflect on her actions and learn from her mistakes may be currently unachievable. Therefore, professionals should be aware of strategies to support her retelling of events, with additional focus on the internal mental states of herself and others. Other strategies around the use of visuals and recording of messages was also suggested, for example, sending voice messages/memos for Clara to listen back to if needed.

The communication profile is a single page with two columns outlining Clara's communication difficulties and strategies to support her, for example:

- **Check you have understood me** by repeating back what you have heard. I might need to say it again.
- **Check I have understood:** Ask me: *'What do you need to do now?'/'Can you tell me what we've talked about?'/'What were we talking about again?'*

I share the profile with all professionals involved in Clara's care, including the Youth Magistrates Court Bench and Police. Two weeks later, after her court hearing, feedback is sent to me:

Value: Justice and fairness

'I can't begin to tell you what a difference this made in Court yesterday! It was amazing, the bench and their approach with her was totally different from her last two experiences.

They communicated with her in a way that she felt reassured by, that she understood and above all she had the confidence to communicate back with them.

...the amount of praise I have received for you and Clara's communication passport has been outstanding, thank you so very much.

Clara, her dad, and the professionals around her have all benefited from your assessment it has been a massive support for us all.'

Approach: Modelling

I arrange follow up visits to Clara to discuss her communication difficulties, to help her understand and to support her narrative skills and mentalisation with the aim of increasing her engagement with the mental health practitioner. Clara goes through cycles of attending sessions, then multiple episodes of being asleep on my arrival to her placement. On some occasions, the staff there tell me she has been up all-night gaming. On others, I am told that Clara was arrested the night before and was being held at the Police Investigation Centre (PIC). At one session, I tell Clara that the sessions would be difficult to justify if she does not attend. I ask if she would like to continue with them and she agrees. When she does attend, she retells stories with the aid of her social media account, and I model how I express my thoughts and feelings, for example, '*I wonder what they thought about that? Maybe they thought...If that was me....*' We then use visual representations of a story arc, with the necessary elements (characters, setting, problem, plan/reaction, action, resolution) and retell a prepared story together. We reflect on how if Clara is unable to tell a story, she might be seen as being unreliable or lying. She nods to show agreement with this. The same narrative strategies are shared with the YJS mental health practitioner to help Clara identify her own emotions, the significance of events and a conclusion. Clara's placement staff and YJS officer report that, when calm and typically 24–48 hours after an event, she is increasingly reflective about her actions and thoughts.

Reflections

Clara's case is complex. Her circumstances are frequently unstable, from moving placements to substance misuse, repeated episodes of maternal rejection, recidivism (her tendency to reoffend) and poor sleep hygiene. For me, it was challenging to know the extent of my role, particularly without clear goal-based interventions for Clara and due to her inconsistency in attending my sessions. I found that my time spent within professional meetings for Clara was effective in being able to help inform expectations, whether that was regarding sitting GCSE exams or taking part in Restorative Justice, where she might struggle to see how her actions have impacted others. I was able to help inform Youth Justice led interventions as well as her mental health practitioner, who, with the information from the report and communication profile, could adapt how they interacted with Clara. Because Clara's situation changed on a weekly and sometimes even hourly basis, I found that working in a multi-disciplinary team allowed me to step in when needed. Sometimes I sat in meetings listening to plans being formed and I could suggest how information could be communicated to Clara. Professionals began to have her communication needs at the forefront of their minds.

Approach: Multi-disciplinary team

Although I did not give a specific diagnosis with a known origin, the over-arching label of SLCN was helpful to discuss with Clara and help her understand why she found learning in school challenging. She accepted this label which I hope replaced the one she previously had – in her own words, but more likely the words of another, that she was *'a retard.'* She has experienced so much in her short life, and the complexity of her history makes it challenging for me to explain why she has these communication difficulties. Where I might have spent an episode of care working on a specific target within a community setting, I found the most impactful intervention was raising awareness of Clara's SLCN and shifting the perspectives of adults around her, and hopefully of Clara herself.

Value: Reassurance

Value: Trust

The reports of Clara's activities and arrests, both inside and outside of her placement, showed a different side to the child who sat with me in sessions and quietly said *'ok'* when I encouraged her to *'give it a go.'* She showed a vulnerability in revealing her difficulties which have plagued her education, and I felt a sense of honour being witness to this. It is hard to think about what different outcome Clara may have had, had her SLCN been identified earlier, but she showed that she has not given up yet.

Questions for reflection and discussion

1. Why might young people with Speech, Language and Communication Needs (SLCN) end up in the Youth Justice System?
2. What are the principles of the Speech and Language Therapist when working with children in YJS?
3. What, if at all, is the role for SLTs in identifying and supporting children with impoverished mentalisation in managing expectations within the wider YJS, Police, education and community?
4. What specific communication skills might SLTs need in order to work with young people in the Youth Justice system?
5. How might SLTs go about encouraging young people to engage fully in their intervention?

Further reading

Mentalization/Theory of Mind: https://manuals.annafreud.org/ambit-static/mentalization

RCSLT (2019). Role of SLT in justice settings: www.rcslt.org/speech-and-language-therapy/where-slts-work/justice/#section-2

RCSLT The Box: A free e-learning tool designed for professionals working in the justice sector: www.rcslt.org/learning/the-box-training/

Youth Justice Resource Hub: https://yjresourcehub.uk/

British Dyslexia Association: www.bdadyslexia.org.uk/

Further information

Theories

Dyslexia: a set of processing difficulties that affect the acquisition of reading and spelling (British Dyslexia Association, 2025).

Narrative competence: being able to understand and produce stories is a key skill in social development as well as educational attainment (Dickinson and McCabe, 2001).

Narrative skills are often an area of significant difficulty for children with SEMH and children who offend and it is this skill that is paramount when navigating the criminal justice system, for example being able to articulate the consequences of one's actions (Cross, 2011).

SLCN (Speech, Language and Communication Needs): it is estimated that over 60% of children in contact with the Youth Justice System have unidentified SLCN (Bryan, 2004).

Theory of mind is our ability to make sense of our own actions and those of others on the basis of intentional mental states such as desires, feelings and beliefs. It is the ability to see ourselves from the outside and others from the inside (Oestergaard Hagelquist and Rasmussen, 2020).

Approaches

Assessing emotion: children with speech, language and communication needs can have difficulties with identifying their own emotions and emotions of others, and may miscategorise others' emotions and, therefore, intentions (Gibson and Toseeb, 2024). This would likely increase their exposure to potentially harmful situations and the risk of Child Criminal Exploitation (CCE).

Case history taking involves gathering information about individuals which can help contextualise their presenting communication difficulties. This includes how long the difficulties have occurred for, any relevant medical information, family history of learning or communication difficulties/disability.

CELF-5 stands for the ***Clinical Evaluation of Language Fundamentals: 5th Ed***. It is a tool for assessing and diagnosing language and communication disorders for individuals aged 5–21 (Wiig, Semel and Secord, 2013).

Child-First: A Child-First Youth Justice System sees children as children, treats them fairly and helps them to build on their strengths so they can make a constructive contribution to society. This will prevent offending and create safer communities with fewer victims: https://yjresourcehub.uk/what-is-child-first/.

Dynamic assessment is a flexible approach to evaluating an individual's communication by looking at their potential rather than at their challenges (Hasson and Joffe, 2007). It can be an appropriate approach in some circumstances, for example, where highlighting an individual's difficulties may cause them to become disengaged.

LfBE (Language for Behaviour and Emotions) is a self-rating tool consisting of thirteen statements covering communication breakdown, understanding and expressing emotions, narrative, inferencing and problem solving. The individual rates each aspect as being: 'easy,' 'tricky sometimes' and 'really tricky' (Branagan, Cross and Parsons, 2020).

Modelling: providing exemplar words, phrases or sentences that the child could use in the future.

Multi-disciplinary team: the often fast paced and complex nature of children in the Youth Justice Service requires a joined up and collaborative approach to ensure plans and intervention are delivered in a timely manner. Collaboration can lead to good outcomes for children with SEMH (Cross, 2011).

Values

Justice and fairness: ensuring an individual is understood in court so their legal outcomes are not unfairly affected by communication barriers.

Reassurance: receiving a diagnosis of Speech, Language and Communication Needs (SLCN) can evoke a range of emotions, both positive and negative. Helping a child understand that this has impacted their education, and that it does not mean that they are incapable of learning, should be done sensitively.

Trust: central to engagement with an individual is their willingness to open up and ensure they can depend on safe, trusted relationships.

References

Branagan, A., Cross, M., and Parsons, S. (2020). ***Language for Behaviour and Emotions***. Routledge. London, UK.

British Dyslexia Association (2025) ***What is Dyslexia?*** www.bdadyslexia.org.uk/

Bryan, K. (2004). Preliminary study of the prevalence of speech and language difficulties in young offenders. ***International Journal of Language and Communication Disorders.*** 39(3), 391–400.

Cross, M. (2011). ***Children with Social, Emotional and Behavioural Difficulties and Communication Problems: There is always a reason.*** Jessica Kingsley Publisher, London UK.

Dickinson, D.K. and McCabe, A. (2001). Bringing it all together: the multiple origins, skills, and environmental supports of early literacy. ***Learning Disabilities Research and Practice***. 16(4), 186–202.

Gibson, J. and Toseeb, U. (2024). ***Developmental Language Disorder and Social-Emotional Development: An Introduction to Theories, Concepts, and Research***. Oxford University Press.

Hasson, N. and Joffe, V. (2007). The case for dynamic assessment in speech and language therapy. ***Child Language Teaching & Therapy.*** 23, 9–25.

Oestergaard Hagelquist, J. and Rasmussen, H. (2020). ***Mentalization in the Family A Guide for Professionals and Parents.*** Routledge.

Wiig, E.H., Semel, E., and Secord, W.A. (2013). ***Clinical Evaluation of Language Fundamentals: 5th Ed (CELF-5)***. Pearson Clinical Assessments.

Case study 4
Ibrahim: 'will I still be able to eat and drink?'

Kirsty Harrison and Neil Coull

Ibrahim's referral

Ibrahim is a 57-year-old, Asian British man. He lives with his wife, Ishra, and their 17-year-old son. He has an older son and daughter, both of whom live nearby and visit regularly with their respective young families. Ibrahim had been a head teacher for many years, but has had to retire on medical grounds, following a diagnosis of Bulbar onset motor neuron disease. Until recently, he has enjoyed a rich social life with hobbies including membership of a running club and socialising with his colleagues at work. His diagnosis has made these activities more difficult for him.

***Theory:* Bulbar onset motor neuron disease**

Ibrahim is under the care of a neurology team, and they have referred him for a Speech and Language Therapy (SLT) assessment following his diagnosis and his reports of changes to his speech and swallowing. In addition, he has lost two stone in weight over the last eight weeks, leading to concerns that he is not meeting his nutritional needs through his current diet. The neurology team is keen to have SLT input to determine the nature of his speech and swallowing difficulties.

Initial impressions

I meet Ibrahim for an outpatient appointment in a hospital to discuss his eating, drinking and swallowing. I want to find out from him what his main concerns are. After introductions, I ask some broad questions to open our discussion.

I begin, *'I've read the referral from your neurologist, but I wanted to hear from you about what brings you here'.*

Ibrahim thinks for a moment and responds, *'I was diagnosed with motor neuron disease about 6 weeks ago. It's*

DOI: 10.4324/9781003668756-6

been a lot to take in, and I keep finding out more about it on the internet. It's all really worrying'. He pauses before continuing, *'I've had to give up work too. I'm mortified about that. I really loved my job, but I just can't do it anymore. It's just all too much'*.

'That does sound like a lot to deal with', I say, *'How are you feeling in yourself?'*

'Just shock, really. My family has been so supportive, but I can tell it's been really hard for them too', he replies.

'It sounds as though it has been a great shock to you all', I say, conscious to mirror some of the language that Ibrahim uses (e.g. *'shock'*). This is in order to build rapport with him. In addition, using words similar to those used by Ibrahim also limit the risk of me adding my interpretation of what he tells me.

Value: Mirroring

As Ibrahim speaks, I am also closely observing his communication, posture, breathing and salivation. I make a number of observations about his speech. Firstly, I notice some hypernasality as he speaks. He is also speaking at a slower rate than is typical and is a bit louder. This suggests to me that he is experiencing Dysarthria.

Theory: Hypernasality

Theory: Dysarthria

Building a picture of Ibrahim's eating and drinking

Having gathered valuable insight into Ibrahim's current knowledge of and feelings towards his diagnosis, I move on to finding out specifically about his eating, drinking and swallowing. I ask, *'Can you tell me about your eating and drinking?'*

'That's all ok. I can eat and drinking everything', he replies, seemingly at odds with what was reported in the referral letter.

Theory: Patient insight

I employ more directed questioning to tease out what was reported, *'Can I ask if you have lost any weight lately?'*

'It's weird, because I have been eating as usual, but these last couple of months I must have lost about two, maybe two and a half stone without even trying', Ibrahim tells me, *'I have even stopped going to my running club, so thought I would put on some weight'*.

'That's a lot of weight to lose in a short space of time', I say, *'But it's fairly typical in MND. There may well be some changes to your swallowing which are contributing to this, but we also know that MND causes changes to your metabolism which adds to the weight loss. Can you tell me about what you're eating in a typical day?'*

Approach: Health coaching

Ibrahim considers this for a moment, *'Well, for breakfast I have toast and coffee'*.

'And how is that going?', I ask.

Approach: Open questions

'I've noticed that I need to put more butter and jam on my toast to get it down', Ibrahim says. He thinks for a moment, *'I'm also drinking my coffee with my toast whereas I just used to drink it at the end'*.

'Mhmm', I say, *'So, it sounds like maybe you're using the coffee to help wash down the toast?'*

Ibrahim consider this, *'Yeah, I think I probably am'*.

'That sounds like a good workaround', I say, *'Are you coughing with your toast and coffee?'*

'Not usually', Ibrahim responds.

I ask, *'Tell me about your lunches at the moment'*.

'I just have something like a soup or daal', he says.

I continue, *'And is that usual for you?'*

'Not really', says Ibrahim, *'I used to have a big sandwich or bagel, but it's hard work now'*.

'In what way?', I ask.

'It kinda doesn't move very easily', he responds.

'Mhmm', I intone, to show I am listening.

Approach: Back-channelling

Ibrahim continues, *'It's hard work actually. Perhaps I am having some difficulties with this that I didn't realise'*.

Further discussion reveals that he has made some additional changes to the types of food he is eating. He reports that he is coughing during most mealtimes which he finds distressing.

Approach: Oro-motor examination

Approach: Oral trials

Next, I carry out an assessment using an oro-motor examination which shows that his tongue and the soft-palate at the back of his mouth are moving with less range and speed than is typical. I ask him to eat food and drink fluids of differing consistencies which reveals further useful information. From my assessment and what Ibrahim tells me, he is showing symptoms of dysphagia. This is characterised by his frequent choking on foods that require a lot of chewing along with weight loss. The oral trial reveals that Ibrahim is able to manage softer foods that are easier to chew and can manage fluids if he takes small sips at a time. These findings inform the advice I give him to make mealtimes safer and more enjoyable for him. Interestingly, he had intuitively known what to do and was avoiding consistencies that he found too difficult. I also encourage him to continue swallowing mouthfuls of drink to help clear any food residue in his mouth after swallowing food, as this seems to be working well for him.

Theory: Dysphagia

Theory: Patient intuition

Addressing the future

Now that I have insight into some of the challenges Ibrahim is facing at mealtimes, I move on to ask him questions about his hopes and fears. I ask him, *'What scares you most?'*

Ibrahim pauses and a concerned look crosses his face, *'Choking'*, he says, *'I'm worried about choking'*.

Theory: Aspiration

We talk about first aid courses that his wife and family can attend and about calling the emergency services for help. I also enquire whether Ibrahim has experienced any chest infections recently without having a cold. This is an important question in determining the risk of aspiration. He tells me that this has not happened. The fact this has not happened is a good sign and suggests that Ibrahim has either been able to clear aspirated material or that food or drink is not reaching this level at present. This will need to be monitored in my future reviews with him as MND can involve respiratory changes which can further complicate swallowing changes.

Next, I ask Ibrahim, *'What are your best hopes for your eating and drinking?'*

Ibrahim says quietly, *'For it to go back to how it used to be.'*

'Mhmm', I acknowledge his response and pause, *'and what are your best hopes for your eating and drinking knowing about your motor neuron disease diagnosis?'*

Approach: Solution Focused Brief Therapy (SFBT)

'You mean knowing it's not going back to normal', he says.

I give a gentle affirmative utterance, *'Mhmm'*.

Ibrahim thinks for a moment, *'I'd like to be able to enjoy family meals again with all the grandkids'*.

'OK...', I say, *'and what would that look like?'*

'Dunno....' he thinks, *'Maybe that I eat a little bit to feel part of it, but that I also get to talk to everyone. I feel quite left out at the moment'*.

'Why is that?' I ask.

'Because I've noticed that when I try to talk and listen when I'm eating, it all goes wrong and that's when I start to cough. So, I either have to eat and not pay attention to anyone, or I just sit there while everyone around me is eating', he says, hopelessly.

Ibrahim has been very insightful and noticed that, for him, eating and drinking alongside conversation are not very compatible.

Theory: Social aspects of mealtimes

'Have you got any ideas about what might help?' I ask.

Ibrahim says, *'I'm not sure really. That's why I have come to see you'.*

'I'm wondering if you had smaller meals more often if that might help?' I say.

'It might take the pressure off a bit', he says, *'Although there would be more to prepare and more washing up. I don't like washing up!'*

'Me neither!', we laugh briefly. I then ask, *'For your family meals, I'm also wondering if it might help if you started your meal a little earlier than everyone else?'*

Value: Humour & humility

Ibrahim looks puzzled, *'How would that help?'*

'It might give you time to focus on your eating and drinking before the conversation starts', I reply, *'You could be finishing your meal as everyone else starts, so you are still eating with everyone. As the conversation gets going, you'll be finishing your meal so might be more able to take part in the conversation'.*

'It might feel a bit weird, but I'll give it a go', he says.

'Yes, it might', I say, *'But it might be worth a try to see if it helps you to be more involved in the family meals that you enjoy so much.'*

I'm attempting to motivate Ibrahim here, reminding him of the key area he would like to change.

Value: Client-centred care

We are nearing the end of the appointment and Ibrahim asks about the future, *'So what is going to happen? With my swallow I mean.'*

'In what respect?' I ask.

'Is it going to get worse?' he says.

'Unfortunately, that is likely, yes. Especially with the type of motor neuron disease you have. It's affecting the throat area first', I say.

Ibrahim looks tearful, *'So what can I do about it?'*

'Sadly, we can't reverse it', I say, *'We don't have a cure for MND yet, so we can't make your swallowing better. But we can look at things that might help your eating and drinking. Some people decide to put a tube in to help with their eating and drinking. Other people choose not to do this.'*

Value: Honesty & integrity

Ibrahim says, *'I don't think that is for me.'*

'Well it's completely your choice', I say, *'It would be good for us to talk about it soon, so you have all the information you need to make the right decision for you. We don't need to talk about this right now though'*.

'OK', he replies.

'Would it be ok if I refer you to a dietitian?' I ask, *'They can help you with getting enough calories and nutrients, so your weight hopefully stabilises a bit'*.

'That would be good, thank you', he says.

I explain, *'They will also be able to help describe the procedure involved with having a tube fitted and talk you through how you might use it.'*

'Wouldn't I just have to use the tube and give up eating and drinking?' Ibrahim says with a look of concern on his face.

'No, not if you didn't want to', I say, reassuringly, *'You can use the tube in different ways. Some people with MND use the tube to get more calories but continue to eat and drink. They find it takes the pressure off having to eat and drink enough and they enjoy eating and drinking smaller amounts of food and drink. So, it doesn't have to be an all or nothing approach'*.

'Oh, I thought it would mean I couldn't eat any more', he says, looking relieved, *'It would be good to find out more about it.'*

'Well, I'll make the referral to the dietitian and if you like, I can come along too and we can discuss all your options', I say, smiling.

'Thank you. That sounds good', says Ibrahim, himself smiling now.

Approach: Interdisciplinary working

I bring the session to a close. Due to the likely fast progressing nature of the disease, a follow-up appointment is arranged with Ibrahim four weeks later so that timely support can be offered.

Reflections

Working with individuals with progressive neurological conditions can require difficult conversations around their inevitable decline over time. In this case, Ibrahim had only recently been diagnosed with MND and understandably this was something that he and his family were coming to terms with. The role of the SLT is to provide advice and support around the aspects of his speech and swallowing affected by the disease. However, as a healthcare professional, there is a wider role to ensure that the needs and concerns of individuals are heard and responded to.

In this initial meeting, I navigated rapport-building with introducing some difficult conversations around future eating and drinking choices. I balanced this with encouraging Ibrahim to share what really mattered to him about the changes to his eating and drinking, building the foundation for collaborative and person-centred intervention planning and paving the way for a productive therapeutic relationship.

Theory: ICF

The International Classification of Functioning (ICF) is a tool used by therapists to consider the individual beyond their disease or impairment. My interview with Ibrahim, for example, considered the wider impact of his swallowing difficulties beyond any physical changes. This was important to consider, as it revealed that what really matters is the impact the changes to his eating and drinking are having on him connecting with his family over mealtimes. Without asking wider questions, it is likely that my advice would not have fully addressed what mattered most to Ibrahim.

I helped Ibrahim to consider his options and to generate solutions for himself. Perhaps I could have stayed with this a little longer than jumping straight in, but I was conscious I wanted to offer suggestions to help develop the rapport between us and so that he might find attending therapy useful.

It was positive that Ibrahim felt able to raise concerns about the future and his changing swallowing. Although not an easy discussion, it is important for SLTs to answer questions honestly and openly. I tried not to overwhelm Ibrahim with lots of information and provided information as he asked for it. I also enabled interdisciplinary working, by seeking his permission to refer him to a dietitian. Decision-making around tube feeding is an individual process, dependent on a range of factors including eating and drinking performance (Labra et al., 2020). Although there is not agreement in healthcare professionals' views about the timing and content of discussions to aid decision-making around tube feeding (White et al., 2024), in my experience a multi-disciplinary discussion between the individual, their family member(s), a dietitian (or gastroenterologist or nutrition specialist nurse) and an SLT can really assist individuals to get the information and facts to help them make an informed decision about tube feeding. In this case, it was helpful to dispel any falsehoods Ibrahim had picked up around tube feeding and to offer him reassurance.

Questions for reflection and discussion

1. In what ways might a diagnosis like MND change an individual's life?
2. What impact might the disease have on Ibrahim's family?
3. How did changes to eating, drinking and swallowing affect Ibrahim's everyday life, beyond getting necessary nutrition and hydration?
4. How would you go about starting difficult conversations with a client?
5. What is the role of an SLT when supporting people with neurodegenerative conditions with eating, drinking and swallowing changes?
6. Why is it beneficial to think of the person beyond simply their illness or diagnosis?

Further reading

Institute of Solution Focused Brief Therapy (SFBT): https://solutionfocused.net/what-is-solution-focused-therapy/

IDDSI (International Diet Description Standardisation Initiative) Framework: www.iddsi.org/standards/framework

MNDA (Motor Neuron Disease Association): www.mndassociation.org/

Yorkston, K. M. (2013). ***Management of speech and swallowing disorders in degenerative diseases***. Pro-Ed.

Further information

Theories

Aspiration is the term used when food or drink travels below the level of the vocal folds inside the larynx. If the food or drink is not cleared by coughing, this can lead to respiratory infections. Commonly chest infections in the absence of a virus can suggest that food or drink has been aspirated.

Bulbar onset motor neuron disease is a rapidly progressing form of motor neuron disease, typically characterised by early signs of speech and swallowing difficulties. There is no current cure, and the symptoms will worsen over time.

Dysarthria: changes in speech, often affecting intelligibility and caused by impairment of muscular control (Duffy, 2019).

Dysphagia: swallowing difficulties caused by impairment of musculature surrounding eating, drinking and swallowing.

Hypernasality: in typical speech, the speaker can rapidly balance the flow of air between the oral cavity (mouth) and nasal cavity (nose) to differentiate speech sounds. Hypernasality refers to excess air flow through the nasal cavity during speech.

ICF (International Classification of Functioning) is a model that enables healthcare professionals to consider the individual holistically as a person rather than just their presentation or illness (World Health Organization, 2001).

Patient insight: it is quite typical for someone with MND to report no problems with their eating and drinking. Whilst they may not have any difficulties, it is also possible that these may not feel like a priority to the individual due to various aspects of life affected by the disease (Lisiecka, Kelly & Jackson, 2019).

Patient intuition: individuals with MND will often intuitively begin to alter what they eat and drink in response to changes to their swallowing abilities (Lisiecka, Kelly & Jackson, 2019).

Social aspects of mealtimes: feelings of connectivity with others and social bonding is associated with mealtimes (Smith, Bryant & Hemsley, 2024). Those with eating and drinking difficulties often cite the loss they feel in the social aspects of eating and drinking.

Approaches

Back-channelling: simple verbal cues, such as agreement, or non-verbal cues, such as nodding, show that we are listening, but encourage the speaker to continue talking.

Health coaching can be employed during patient consultations to empower individuals with knowledge about their illness.

Interdisciplinary working: drawing on the skills and knowledge of a wide range of health and medical professionals is important in the effective management of neurological diseases such as MND.

Open questions: enable individuals to answer freely. Alternately, closed questions, for example, those requiring 'yes/no' answers, can be helpful in narrowing the focus.

Oral trials: assessing individuals by using food and fluids of different consistencies can determine the safest options for eating and drinking. The IDDSI (International Diet Description Standardisation Initiative) Framework provides a standardised approach for Speech and Language Therapists to use (Cichero et al., 2017).

Oro-motor examination looks at the appearance and movement of different parts of the mouth and throat in order to determine the nature of the individual's speech and swallowing difficulties.

Solution Focused Brief Therapy (SFBT) can help people to articulate what matters most about an issue they are experiencing (Burns & Northcott, 2022). In turn, as an SLT, you can use this to guide intervention ensuring it is meaningful and person-centred.

Values

Client-centred care planning treatment is based on the individual's priorities and needs. This is likely to be more relevant and motivating to them.

Honesty and integrity are key attributes of the healthcare professional's role to ensure patient concerns are addressed. This may mean addressing difficult or challenging questions, and as such, sensitivity is needed in terms of how these concerns are addressed.

Humour and humility, when used appropriately, can be key attributes of a therapist's role that can help to keep healthcare interactions grounded.

Mirroring is an approach to communicating in which the listener subtly echoes the verbal and non-verbal behaviours of the speaker in order to show empathy and connection with others. It can be a useful tool for healthcare professionals to build rapport.

References

Burns, K., & Northcott, S. (2022). ***Working with solution focused brief therapy in healthcare settings: A practical guide.*** Routledge.

Cichero, J. A., Lam, P., Steele, C. M., Hanson, B., Chen, J., Dantas, R. O., Duivestein, J., Kayashita, J., Lecko, C., Murray, J., & Pillay, M. (2017). Development of international terminology and definitions for texture-modified foods and thickened fluids used in dysphagia management: The IDDSI framework. ***Dysphagia, 32***(2), 293–314. https://doi.org/10.1007/s00455-016-9758-y

Duffy, J. R. (2019). ***Motor speech disorders: Substrates, differential diagnosis, and management*** (4th ed.). Elsevier.

Labra, J., Hogden, A., Power, E., James, N., & Flood, V. M. (2020). Gastrostomy uptake in motor neurone disease: A mixed-methods study of patients' decision making. ***BMJ Open, 10***(2), e034751. https://doi.org/10.1136/bmjopen-2019-034751

Lisiecka, D., Kelly, H., & Jackson, J. (2019). How do people with motor neurone disease experience dysphagia? A qualitative investigation of personal experiences. ***Disability and Rehabilitation*, *43***(4), 479–488. https://doi.org/10.1080/09638288.2019.1630487

Smith, R., Bryant, L., & Hemsley, B. (2024). 'I only eat because I have to—to live': The impacts of dysphagia on quality of life from the perspectives of people with dysphagia, supporters of people with dysphagia and allied health professionals. ***International Journal of Language & Communication Disorders*, *59***(5), 1966–1980. https://doi.org/10.1111/1460-6984.12986

White, S., O'Cathain, A., Halliday, V., Bradburn, M., & McDermott, C. J. (2024). Supporting people with motor neuron disease (MND) to make decisions about gastrostomy feeding tube placement: A survey of UK healthcare professionals' practice and beliefs. ***Amyotrophic Lateral Sclerosis and Frontotemporal Degeneration*, *25***(3–4), 290–298. https://doi.org/10.1080/21678421.2024.2314061

World Health Organization. (2001). ***International classification of functioning, disability and health (ICF).*** www.who.int/standards/classifications/international-classification-of-functioning-disability-and-health

Part 2

Working with significant others – family, friends and carers

Case study 5
Safwan: supporting families with early communication development

Mst. Meherunnessa Mim

Background and referral

I meet Safwan and his mother by chance, when I visit a Specialist Educational School to collect data for my research. On the first day of my visit there, Safwan's mother approaches knowing my Speech and Language Pathology (SLP) background from the class teacher who suggested she talk to me about Safwan's speech concerns. We have an almost fifteen-minute conversation where she shares how Safwan seems different from others and can not talk at all, how difficult it is for her to understand his needs. She then asks if I will be able to help Safwan to develop his language ability, where my office is, and how she can book a session. With my guidance, she is able to book an appointment with me so that I can formally assess Safwan to identify his receptive and expressive language deficits, communication difficulties and determine the appropriate diagnosis. At the first session both of his parents are present, and his mother shares: *'Safwan was diagnosed with* DS *immediately after birth. We were in shock and felt helpless as we had no idea how to help him. Both of us and our other family members initially thought it will cure over time.'*

Approach: Assessment

Theory: Down's Syndrome (DS)

Last year, Safwan's parents decided to admit him to a preschool, but the preschools in Dhaka, Bangladesh go through admission processes including tasks such as following simple commands, identifying basic shapes or colours, telling the names of their father, mother and themselves when asked. As Safwan could not do these things, he got rejected by at least five preschools. His mother was totally devastated at that time, and she then reached out for help to one of her friends who has a cousin with DS. Her friend suggested admitting him to a special school.

Approach: Referral

DOI: 10.4324/9781003668756-8

His father adds, *'We admitted him to a nearby special school, but he could not cope there either. After one year of trying, his special educator suggested us to seek SLT support along with special education for his development.'*

Approach: Speech and Language Therapy

Approach: Speech and Language Therapist (SLT) role

They hope that their child will be able to communicate and lead a normal life. They do not have any idea what to expect from me and how the Speech and Language Therapist (SLT) will be helpful for Safwan.

Assessment findings

I complete Safwan's assessment in three sessions as I want to assess him in his most natural environment, to conduct a comprehensive assessment.

The first session includes an interview with his parents about his background information and medical history.

His mother shares,

'I was completely healthy during my pregnancy and there were no major complications during birth. I did not know or was told by the doctors about his condition while I was pregnant. We have no family history of any kind of communication disorders.'

His father adds, *'I was a late talker according to my family members. But it was not taken very seriously in my family.'*

Safwan's vision is normal according to his medical documentations. The co-occurrence of hearing disorders with DS is quite a common phenomenon and almost 80% of people with DS have some form of hearing disorder (Shott, 2000). However, Safwan does not have any hearing disorder, and this is diagnosed by an audiologist.

I identify some restricted behaviors and repetitive motor movements of Safwan like his continuous hand flapping. Surprisingly, he does not seem to have neologism. He does not have any history of epilepsy and is not on any medication currently.

His mother shares,

'Safwan gets very hyper when he does not get noodles, or if any changes happen in his daily routine, and if someone forces him to communicate. He used to eat all kinds of foods but suddenly at the age of three stopped eating anything but noodles. Moreover, his noodles must be prepared with a watery and soup like texture. Otherwise, he won't eat. At first, I tried to force him to eat other foods, but his extreme meltdown over the foods stopped me from trying.'

'What are the relieving factors you notice or what keeps him calm?' I ask.

'I will say to be alone, getting pictures or toys of animal figures and getting breaks from his tasks', his mother replies.

In the second session, I observe him in the playground and in the classroom, with his peers and teachers to find out his most natural behavior and make comprehensive assessments.

Finally in the third session, I interact with him and try to involve him in some tasks. On each session or communication with him I do not wear an apron, which is a widespread practice of SLTs in Bangladesh, because his mother suggested that he can get uncomfortable and confused as he is only familiar with doctors or people at hospitals wearing one.

The assessment of pre-verbal skills

In my observation, Safwan avoids eye contact and does not respond when called by his name. He is not interested in others around him, even in the playground of the school he is playing alone with his toy animal.

Theory: Pre-verbal skills

Safwan's attention is very restricted, and he loves to be busy with only one object for a long period of time. He can point but sometimes fails to point because of indifference. He does not request at all but has a minimum understanding of someone requesting him to do some tasks (mostly tasks that are previously practiced or are part of his routine).

His reasoning abilities are absent, however, choice making is spontaneous, for example, he always chooses noodles over any food items, and animal figure toys for playing. Turn-taking skills are present but not spontaneous.

He has a limited understanding of cause and effect. While observing him at school I witnessed a very surprising incident. Safwan was in his own world, as always, but suddenly I saw him packing his bag as soon as he noticed a man who was waiting outside. Later I found out that man was his driver, who always picks him up from school for home. This incident showed that he has anticipation of organizing his bag and going back home.

The assessment of receptive language skills

Theory: Receptive language skills

Safwan can identify bottle, book, bag and pencil, and is able to point to these objects when asked. He has a good comprehension of some food utensils (spoon, glass, bottle) and can identify them from pictures.

When I show him pictures of his school and home along with other pictures, he can identify them successfully. I also have printed pictures of his mother, father, sister, brother and class teacher, and he can identify them. He shows an excessive interest in animals and can identify common animals (dog, cat, cow, duck, horse, lion, tiger). He shows his hand, leg, eye and head when asked.

When I give a command to stand, he stands up but does not wait for the command to sit. He sits immediately after he gets up. He responds well to questions like: "what?" and "which one?"

He understands some adjectives in Bengali like good, beautiful, less and more. He understands verbs like eating, going, sleeping and walking.

He remains silent and non-responsive when I ask him yes/no questions. He does not have any idea of the question "Where?" There is a total absence of understanding of pronouns, and he has a problem understanding two key-word sentences, commands, directions and questions.

The assessment of expressive language skills

Theory: Expressive language skills

Safwan can imitate me when I say **/a/ /o/** but cannot imitate **/i/ /u/**. He cannot produce any consonants. He cannot name any objects. He does not request at all, neither by gesture nor speech.

The assessment of non-verbal communication

Theory: Non verbal communication

Theory: Theory of Mind

He can point to some single-word objects and pictures, and copies basic Bengali gestures (salam and bye), which he learned after joining the Specialist Educational School. His posture seems normal, but he walks slowly and has bent shoulders while standing, which is a common feature of children with DS. He refuses to shake hands or give a high-five. He cannot express his feelings using expressions; he does not smile at all, but cries when he is forced to do something that he does not want to do. His Theory of Mind (ToM) is also not developed as per his mother and he tries to hurt people, through scratching and biting, during meltdowns.

The assessment of cognitive skills

Theory: Cognitive skills

Safwan avoids cognitive tasks in my sessions. Some of his activities (organising bag before going home, bringing out tiffin box during tiffin time, and following daily routines) make me think that he has the ability to reason but after assessing properly, I understand that those activities are just his daily habits, which he adheres to.

The assessment of articulators

Theory : Articulators

Theory: Hypotonia

In the assessment I find hypotonia of the lips, tongue, jaw and cheeks. He has a protruding tongue, which is the cause of his poor lip closure. He has limited ability to elevate, retract or lateralize the tongue, which creates difficulties in copying the lip and tongue's movements.

Theory: Autism Spectrum Disorder (ASD)

Theory: Comorbid disorders

Theory: DSM-5

The prevalence of Autism Spectrum Disorder (ASD) in individuals with DS is found by researchers with the rate of 5% to 39% (Capone et al., 2005; Lowenthal et al., 2007). Children with comorbid DS-ASD display significant expressive and receptive language delays and impairments (Ward & Sanoudaki, 2021). ASD is the reason Safwan is not interested in communicating with others at all, and he never felt that he needed to express himself through speech or language. Mostly children with DS only demonstrate differences in social and expressive language skills when compared to their DS-ASD peers (Sultan et al., 2020). I find Safwan's expressive language skills severely impaired. For some individuals with DS, a pattern of atypical social behaviors, along with known cognitive and linguistic impairments, can mark the comorbidity of ASD (Chapman & Hesketh, 2000). Safwan does not seem to notice people, is less likely to communicate, shows resistance in group activity, is easily startled at loud sounds and flaps his hand continuously. Using the DSM-5 (American Psychiatric Association, 2013) diagnostic criteria, I identify that he meets the criteria for ASD with Level 3 severity.

Intervention design

Approach: Therapy

Value: Client-centered therapy

Value: Parental inclusion

As a Speech and Language Therapist (SLT) I always aim to provide reasonable and client-centered therapy. All my goals are discussed with Safwan's parents, especially with his mother. I make sure the parents understand that therapy outcomes are inherently probabilistic rather than deterministic. My long-term goals are focused on developing his pre-verbal skills; developing receptive language skills; improving coordination of articulators; and developing expressive language skills and social communication skills.

The following short-term goals are targeted to achieve the long-term goals:

1. Improving the strength and coordination of the lip, tongue and jaw.
2. Improving eye contact, attention, pointing, gesture, turn-taking, reasoning and social greeting skills.

3. In the expressive language skill, goals include increasing the percentage of Bengali sounds production at phoneme, word, phrase and sentence level.
4. The receptive language short-term goal is to develop his vocabulary of more daily life objects, increasing the understanding of body parts, basic colors, shapes, pronouns, ten basic adjectives, basic verbs, yes/no questions, prepositions, one-word sentences, two-keyword sentences including commands, and questions simultaneously.

Though the short-term goals seem a lot, I just tried to point out all the things I need to work on sequentially. I plan sessional goals, depending on Safwan's performance. I will try to include four activities (at least one from each part). This is how my sessions mostly look:

Me, "*Salam*" (Muslim greetings)

Mostly Safwan gestures Salam.

Safwan recently showed interest in bubbles which is a great opportunity for me to encourage some pre-verbal skills like eye contact and attention.

Then I move on to some receptive language development tasks, such as picture exchange. He can currently identify one picture when given two options of daily object pictures. I am trying to introduce three options, but he still gets confused when presented with three pictures and is asked to pick one. We are continuing to work on this.

Then I work on his expressive language, and I am trying not to force him to say anything; we just do rhymes together. He mostly does not show any interest in saying anything, but he now enjoys his rhyming sessions with me. He gets very calm and sometimes imitates my gestures which I do repeatedly in the rhyme like clapping. He sometimes copies some syllables too.

After that I focus on the Oro-motor exercises (OME). I keep this stage for the last ten minutes of the session because

Approach: Oro-motor exercises (OME)

Safwan gets very irritated while practicing OME. I am trying to find out ways to make him comfortable and make this more playful and enjoyable.

Safwan is taking two sessions (each consisting of 45 minutes) in a week, which is not enough for his development. Therefore, I always include his mother in the therapy sessions so that she can learn the tasks and help Safwan to practice at home.

I referred his parents to get an appointment of an Occupational Therapist as he has attention and sensory issues.

Outcome measurement

For outcome measurement I use a weekly probe sheet. I document one in my session and provide one sheet to his mother so that the daily target can be measured. After one week his mother and I go through both sheets and plan the goal of the next week and tasks for the next sessions. If the percentage of correct responses is more than 75–80% then the weekly session is marked as a successful session and we move to the next level. Otherwise, I target the least achieved goal and continue working on it.

Initial outcome

After three months of taking sessions and continuous practices, Safwan is now able to utter /i/, /e/, /u/ vowels separately with only visual cue and pa, ba syllables with tactile cues. His jaw and lip muscle strength and movement have improved. He learned to blow, however still cannot forcefully blow. Safwan now maintains eye contact while I blow bubbles or take his favorite toys and pictures to my nose. His turn-taking skills also improved, for example, taking turns to match the puzzles or ball throwing activity.

His pointing skills have also improved. In session, when I command *"Show Ammu (mother)"* he points to his mother. Then *"Show Aunty (Me/SLT)"* he points to me. After that I command, *"Show Safwan"* and he points to himself. I try to change the directions sequences to make it generalised and not something restricted. However, his reasoning and social greeting skills have not improved at all.

In the part of receptive language skill, Safwan seems to be doing better. His outcome measurement score also increased in receptive language skills. When asked, he can now identify and give for 20 daily object items correctly. He can also match those 20 daily objects to their pictures.

His mother shared, '*He now points to his water bottle every time he is thirsty, wears shoes, and points to the door when he wants to go outside.*'

This is a milestone in his learning process. Understanding of colours and shapes is still underdeveloped.

He still does not understand pronouns so we are now only trying to teach him the nouns; most commands are given using nouns instead of pronouns. His understanding of two-key word sentences and commands is not developed yet.

Reflections

When I started working with Safwan, the most challenging task for me was to convince his parents to continue his therapy. In Bangladesh, the field of SLT is not well known by the general population. People still think people with DS and/or ASD are mentally retarded and there is no way to help them. On the other hand, some people tend to be superstitious and unaware of the helpfulness of early intervention. His mother spends most of her time with Safwan. She shared that some of the family members suggested waiting and being patient with Safwan and not to seek help, as his father was a late speaker, according to them. Even after starting the therapy sessions, his parents were unaware of what to expect. His father asked on the first session how long it will take or how many sessions will be needed for Safwan to be verbal. Therefore, dealing with the parents, convincing them of realistic goal setting, was difficult for me. However, I managed to convince his parents, mostly his mother. I am now trying to convince them

Theory: Early intervention

for Alternative and Augmentative Communication (AAC). Safwan will be able to communicate better if he gets access to AAC, as his receptive language skills are getting better, and we will try to introduce Picture Exchange Communication System (PECS).

Questions for reflection and discussion

1. Why is early diagnosis and intervention important for children with communication disorders?
2. Why is the diagnosis of comorbidity necessary when a child has comorbid communication disorders?
3. How can the referral process help the parents of a child with communication disorders?
4. How might caregivers' or parents' traditional beliefs or superstitions influence their perceptions and support of a child with communication disorders?
5. Why is explaining therapy goals and plans to parents necessary?
6. How can an SLT include parents and other professionals in their therapy programs?

Further reading

Down Syndrome–Autism Connection: https://ds-asd-connection.org/

Down Syndrome International: www.ds-int.org/

Autism Speaks: www.autismspeaks.org/

Hamner, T., Hepburn, S., Zhang, F., Fidler, D., Rosenberg, C. R., Robins, D. L., & Lee, N. R. (2020). Cognitive profiles and autism symptoms in comorbid Down syndrome and autism spectrum disorder. ***Journal of Developmental & Behavioral Pediatrics***, *41*(3), 172–179. https://doi.org/10.1097/DBP.0000000000000745

Unnerstall, T. (2020). ***A New Course: A Mother's Journey Navigating Down Syndrome and Autism***. Down Syndrome Dallas.

Further information

Theories

Articulators are the speech organs involved in the production of speech. The muscle strength, coordination and proper functioning of lip, teeth, tongue, jaw and palate are particularly important for speech production.

Autism Spectrum Disorder (ASD) is a neurodevelopmental condition. Individuals with ASD have persistent deficits in verbal social communication and show restricted and repetitive behavior, interests and activities (American Psychiatric Association, 2013).

Cognitive skills are those higher level processes involving memory, attention, problem-solving, reasoning and planning

Comorbid disorders is a term used where two or more distinct disorders or conditions are simultaneously present in an individual. For example, a child with DS may also have ASD or ADHD. This is particularly important to identify if the child has any comorbid disorders for his/her development.

Down's Syndrome (DS) is a genetic disorder resulting from either an additional copy of chromosome 21 or a complete extra copy of it, occurring in about one out of every 1,100 live births (World Health Organization, 2017). This leads to developmental and intellectual difficulties and causes speech and language disorders.

DSM-5 or ***Diagnostic and Statistical Manual of Mental Disorders, 5th Edition***, is used to define and evaluate mental and developmental disorders. This book is published by the American Psychiatric Association and is widely acceptable for guidance and documented diagnosis of different mental and developmental disorders. Clinicians can rely on this book for their assessment and diagnosis.

Early intervention refers to the early assessment, diagnosis and therapy initiation for young children with speech and language disorders to support optimal growth and learning. This focuses on identifying and addressing challenges in infancy or preschool years when the brain is most adaptable.

Expressive language skills indicate the production of language, which consists of the ability to convey thoughts, ideas and feelings. Human interaction or communication is important and if anyone faces difficulties in expressing themselves that will affect all aspects of their life.

Hypotonia is the reduced muscle tone that affects the functioning of the muscles. This is also called floppy muscle tone. It can create speech problems along with feeding and swallowing issues.

Non-verbal communication is communicating through facial expressions, gestures, posture and body language without speech and language.

Pre-verbal skills are the skills that play a key role in the language development of a child that emerges before spoken language. It includes eye contact, joint attention, turn-taking, babbling and gestures.

Receptive language skills are the ability to comprehend and process language. If a child has delayed receptive language skills that will hamper the growth of vocabulary and overall expressive language skills. Therefore, focusing on the receptive language skills in the therapy planning is particularly important.

Theory of Mind (ToM) is the understanding of others' thoughts, beliefs and emotions. It enables people to recognize that others may hold different perspectives from their own. Difficulties with ToM are common in ASD, often leading to social misunderstandings or challenges in predicting others' behaviours.

Approaches

Assessment is a structured process of gathering information about a client's communication abilities and disabilities. It can be both formal and informal. As Bangladesh is still a developing country where SLT is not widely popular, mostly clinicians still use informal approaches of assessment as the formal assessment tools are very costly.

Oro-motor exercises (OME) are a set of oral exercises or activities to improve strength and functioning of oral muscles. These are especially useful for clients with hypotonia, dysarthria or articulation difficulties.

Referral is the process of ensuring children receive timely input from other healthcare services, as required. In cases such as this, other services may include the following: Occupational Therapists, ENT surgeons, pediatric doctors, audiologists, psychologists and special educators. Ideally, these different professionals would work together to support the individual.

Speech and Language Therapy is the service provided to clients with speech and language difficulties or swallowing problems. The professionals are known as Speech and Language Therapists.

Speech and Language Therapist (SLT) role includes responsibilities like assessment, diagnosis and therapy for clients with speech-language and swallowing disorders. They also play a key role in advocacy, awareness-raising and research in the field of communication disorders. The SLT also counsels the parents if needed to help them understand and accept the way of therapy, guiding families toward realistic goals while supporting their hopes for progress.

Therapy is the individualised intervention planning for clients with communication disorders based on their assessments. Before initiating therapy, SLT should design goals that are SMART: specific, measurable, achievable, relevant and time bound.

Values

Client-centered therapy means tailoring intervention to the client's individual needs, preferences and goals.

Parental inclusion is ensuring parents' participation in the therapy sessions, goal setting and home practice; prioritising parents' advice to support and promote their child's needs. Parental involvement strengthens outcomes, fosters collaboration between therapist and family and creates a supportive environment for the child's learning.

References

American Psychiatric Association. (2013). ***Diagnostic and statistical manual of mental disorders*** (5th ed.). American Psychiatric Publishing.

Capone, G. T., Grados, M. A., Kaufmann, W. E., Bernad-Ripoll, S., & Jewell, A. (2005). Down syndrome and comorbid autism-spectrum disorder: Characterization using the aberrant behavior checklist. ***American Journal of Medical Genetics Part A, 134***(4), 373–380.

Chapman, R. S., & Hesketh, L. J. (2000). Behavioral phenotype of individuals with Down syndrome. ***Mental Retardation and Developmental Disabilities Research Reviews***, ***6***(2), 84–95.

Lowenthal, R., Paula, C. S., Schwartzman, J. S., Brunoni, D., & Mercadante, M. T. (2007). Prevalence of pervasive developmental disorder in Down's syndrome. ***Journal of Autism and Developmental Disorders***, ***37***(7), 1394–1395.

Shott, S. R. (2000). Down syndrome: Common pediatric ear, nose, and throat problems. ***Down Syndrome Quarterly***, ***5***(2), 1–6.

Sultan, A., Juneja, A., & Bhaskar, S. (2020). Co-morbidity of down syndrome with autism spectrum disorder: Dental implications. ***Journal of Oral Biology and Craniofacial Research***, ***10***(2), 146–148.

Ward, R., & Sanoudaki, E. (2021). Bilingualism in children with a dual diagnosis of Down syndrome and Autism Spectrum Disorder. ***Clinical Linguistics & Phonetics***, ***35***(7), 663–689.

World Health Organization. (2017). Genomic Resource Centre: Genes and human disease. ***Genes and Chromosomal Diseases***.

Case study 6
Adrianna: language difficulties or language differences?

Lily Basley

Adrianna's referral

Adrianna was referred to the community paediatric Speech and Language Therapy (SLT) team by her class teacher, who raised concerns about her functional use of language and social communication skills. Adrianna is bilingual as she has been consistently exposed to English in school and Romanian at home.

Before this referral, Adrianna had received 12 weeks of intervention from the school's in-house communication team. Their work was guided by the WellComm assessment. Based on this, Adrianna took part in twice weekly one-to-one intervention sessions using activities from the WellComm's 'Big Book of Ideas'. She also participated in twice-weekly 'Box Time'. While Adrianna made some progress, her follow-up WellComm screening still placed her in the red category, signalling the need for specialist input.

Approach: WellComm assessment

Approach: Box Time

At the time of this referral, Adrianna was also awaiting assessment as part of the Education, Health and Care Plan (EHCP) process. She had also been referred to the Neurodevelopmental Service (NDS) by the Community Paediatric Team for further investigation into possible neurodiversity. As part of that pathway, the NDS requested a report based on DSM-5 criteria from our community SLT service.

Approach: EHCP

Approach: NDS

Theory: DSM-5 (Diagnostic and Statistical Manual of Mental Disorders (5th edition)

Observing Adrianna

I meet Adrianna for the first time in her classroom and observe her during free play. My aim is to gain a naturalistic understanding of her functional communication skills and how she interacts with her peers in an unstructured setting.

Approach: Observation

Theory: Functional communication

DOI: 10.4324/9781003668756-9

Theory: Imaginative play

During this observation, I note that Adrianna mostly plays alone. She engages in imaginative play with a baby doll – soothing it, putting it to bed, and talking to it. When other children attempt to interrupt her play or remove toys she is using, she protests appropriately by shouting '*no*' and pushing them away.

Functionally, Adrianna uses simple sentences to communicate. For example, during my observation, Adrianna approaches me and says, '*Teacher, he needs bandage*', while pointing to a peer who appears to have a cut on his knee. This suggests to me that she can generate short, meaningful utterances to meet her communicative needs and that she has an awareness of the needs of others. However, she does not recognise that I am an unfamiliar adult and generalises the role of 'teacher' to any adult within the setting. I also notice throughout our interaction that she frequently echoes the language and intonation patterns of my speech that I use.

Meeting Adrianna's teacher

Following my observation, I speak with Adrianna's class teacher to gather further information.

I begin by saying, '*I just wanted to follow up after my observation and get a bit of information from you as an adult who has been working with Adrianna for the last 6 months. Would you say this is typical of Adrianna's presentation in class?*'

'*Mostly yes*', the teacher confirms, '*she can follow the classroom routine well. But if she chooses not to, she'll just sit there with her eyes closed and disengage*'.

'*Ok thank-you*', I say, and move on to my next question, '*Can you tell me a bit more about her use of language? How does she get her wants and needs across?*'

The teacher reflects for a moment. '*Well*', she says, '*She does approach adults to initiate contact or make requests, usually using single words like "drink" or "toilet". If she can't say what she wants, she'll take your hand and lead you to it instead.'*

I nod and continue, *'and is there anything else you have noticed about her communication skills?'*

The teacher considers this question, pausing momentarily. *'Yes'*, she says, *'she often repeats what she hears – like an echo, and sometimes she does it using what sounds like an American accent.'*

Assessing Adrianna informally

After the classroom observation, I carry out an informal one-to-one assessment with Adrianna. This is conducted in English, in a quiet room separate from the classroom. My approach is based on Blank Levels. I observe that Adrianna only responds accurately to Blank Level 1 questions, for example, naming items recently or directly in front of her. Typically, a child of her age should be able to demonstrate competency at Blank Level 4, which highlights the significant difficulties Adrianna was presenting with in her understanding of language.

Approach: Informal assessment

Theory: Blank Levels

I ask Adrianna to describe photographs of people performing actions. She predominantly uses nouns, for example, she says *'chair'* when asked to name the action, *'sitting'*. I provide prompts to try and support her to elicit the correct action word such as providing sentence frames: *'the girl is... [sitting]'*. However, she does not respond to these prompts. Throughout the assessment, I notice that Adrianna avoids making eye contact with me and does not engage in any reciprocal conversation when I ask about her day at school or her interests.

As English is an additional language for Adrianna, I arrange a follow-up assessment conducted in Romanian with the support of a professional interpreter. I am keen to find out whether her language difficulties are only present in her use of English. I meet with the interpreter prior to the appointment for a briefing.

Value: Accessibility

I start by gauging the interpreter's knowledge of my role by asking, *'Thank-you for joining me today to support this session. Have you worked with a children's Speech and Language Therapist before?'*

The interpreter replies, *'No, I mostly work in the court services with adults.'*

I then explain the purpose of the session, *'That's ok. I will explain what we're going to do in the session. We will have time for questions too. We are going to be looking at Adrianna's understanding and use of Romanian. Adrianna is 6 years old – there are concerns regarding her use and understanding of language. She is also undergoing assessment for Autism Spectrum Condition. Therefore, there might be differences in her social communication skills during the session. I have already assessed her in English, so I am now trying to gather whether her difficulties are across both languages. I would like to speak as little English as possible during the session so that Adrianna understands that we are focusing on Romanian. I have prepared these pictures, and I just need you to ask these questions in Romanian. Could you check that these questions translate appropriately into Romanian – or if we need to tweak them if not?'*

After reviewing the resources, the interpreter confirms '*Yes, these are fine*'.

I then explain the information I need recorded during the session, *'I would like you to ask and record her answers in Romanian. If Adrianna replies in English, please ask her to reply in Romanian. If she doesn't, continue asking the rest of the questions in Romanian and I will record the English answers.'*

The interpreter confirms that she does not have any further questions, so Adrianna then joins us for the session. During this session, Adrianna can answer Blank Level 1 questions when asked in Romanian. However, she responds only in English even though the interpreter encourages her to reply in Romanian. Adrianna is able to echo answers modelled in Romanian but does not respond spontaneously in the language. However, this suggests that she can understand Romanian.

Working with Adrianna's mother

Following the assessment sessions, I meet with Adrianna's mother in person to share my findings. This session is also supported by a professional interpreter, as Adrianna's mother does not speak English.

I start by introducing the purpose of my assessment: *'Thank-you for joining me today. I was asked to assess Adrianna's communication and social interaction skills as part of the NDS process for the assessment of Autism Spectrum Condition'*. I pause to allow the interpreter to translate before continuing, *'I carried out an observation in class, spoke to her class teacher and carried out informal assessment with Adrianna'*, I pause frequently to give time to both the interpreter and Adrianna's mother, *'I found that she has difficulties in engaging in imaginative play with others, building friendships, maintaining eye contact, and sharing interests with others. I also identified that Adrianna has challenges in her understanding and use of language in both English and Romanian.'*

Adrianna's mother reports via the interpreter, *'My daughter only uses Romanian at home when she doesn't know the English word for something. Otherwise, she only speaks in English. So, I don't have concerns regarding her use of Romanian as she does not properly speak it. I also feel that Adrianna is not Autistic. It feels that professionals here (England) are too quick to diagnose children. When she is at home, she plays with our neighbour's children all the time.'*

'I understand what you are saying', I use in a reassuring tone, *'children can have different presentations in different environments and that is why my contribution is just one part of the diagnostic process. Your observations of her at home are also important in helping us to understand Adrianna's needs and will help with a diagnosis'*.

We then discuss next steps and the proposed plan for support. I explain, *'In my report, I have recommended that Adrianna receives one-to-one intervention from the school's communication team and classroom staff, focusing on targeted areas in English. I would also like to show you how to work on some activities in Romanian at home.'*

Adrianna's mother advises, *'She never wants to play with me at home. If I try to join her play, she will walk away. She spends most of her time playing on her tablet.'*

I asked, *'I can appreciate that, but would you consider understanding and use of Romanian to be an important part of Adrianna's identity?'*

She admitted, *'no not really – she only ever speaks English and goes to an English school.'*

I explain, *'Adrianna is exposed to sufficient English in school. However, Romanian is just as important and a big part of her cultural heritage – it is not possible for school staff to support Romanian language development, so I need you to support her to preserve her understanding and use of Romanian at home. Otherwise, she may be at risk of losing it entirely. You only speak Romanian, and I imagine you have other family members who do not speak English – it's important that Adrianna can communicate with them to maintain those family links. I acknowledge that it can be difficult to work with children on structured activities at home – especially after a day at school. However, I would like you to work on Blank Level 2 questions with Adrianna and these types of questions can be built into everyday routines and interactions as opposed to doing a "sit-down" formal task.'*

We then review translated activity ideas and resources focused on developing Adrianna's understanding of Blank Level 2 questions in Romanian. Adrianna's mother agrees to try and build these questions into home life.

Next steps

Following this meeting, I write a report which I share with the EHCP coordinator, the school, the NDS team and

Adrianna's parents. Adrianna's care is then transferred back to the school team to allow them to continue working towards the identified targets within the school environment in English and with parents supporting Romanian at home. Two terms later, Adrianna has been re-referred to the service, having successfully achieved her initial targets. This is positive. She continues to require ongoing support but is clearly making progress.

Reflections

Working with parents: challenges and opportunities

One of the biggest challenges I encountered in this case was supporting parental understanding of the importance of continuing intervention and communication in the home language. A key responsibility for Speech and Language Therapists working with multilingual families is to help them understand the potential risks of language attrition when home languages are not actively supported. Children attending English-speaking educational settings are typically exposed to sufficient English throughout the school day to support both development and maintenance of the language. Therefore, it is not only appropriate but preferable for languages other than English (LOTE) to be prioritised and nurtured in the home environment.

In my experience, some parents express concern that they should only promote English at home because it is perceived as *'the language of education.'* However, research consistently demonstrates that developing a strong foundation in any language gives the child the necessary skills to learn additional languages. It is therefore imperative that parents speak to their children in the language they are most confident and competent in speaking to support the child to develop those skills.

From a cultural perspective, maintaining the home language is vital for a child's sense of identity and belonging. It enables them to connect with their cultural heritage and ensures they can communicate with extended family members, including older relatives who may not speak English (Inan & Harris, 2025).

An important aspect of my role involved supporting Adrianna's parents as they navigated the process of understanding and accepting her neurodiversity. For many families, receiving a diagnosis can trigger a complex emotional response, often involving a period of adjustment or grief as they reconcile their expectations with a new understanding of their child's needs.

Cultural differences and expectations

In my experience, families from certain cultural backgrounds may view autism primarily through a medical lens, perceiving it as a condition to be '*fixed*.' This belief can lead some to pursue extensive, and often unnecessary, medical investigations. This can include international consultations and diagnostic procedures as they search for a potential cure. Such cultural and societal influences can significantly shape a family's response to a diagnosis and may present additional challenges in their understanding of autism.

Although it is important to recognise and validate parents' feelings with regards to the differences in a child's presentation between settings, it is my professional responsibility to contribute towards the NDS process and to explain my findings to parents in relation to the diagnostic criteria. Despite their reservations, Adrianna's parents had provided their consent for the initial referral and were engaging with professionals.

Shifting perspectives on neurodiversity

Value: Neuroaffirming practice

In recent years, the field of SLT has been moving towards adopting more neuroaffirming approaches in supporting individuals with autism. Historically, the focus was often on modifying the individual's behaviour to fit neurotypical expectations. However, there is now a growing recognition of the importance of adapting environments and communication approaches to better support and respect the unique needs and strengths of neurodivergent individuals (RCSLT, n.d.b). Therefore, in my practice, I regularly make indirect recommendations to support settings and staff in adopting a more neuroaffirming approach.

Raising a neurodiverse child can put parents under additional strain. Research has recognised that parents of children with autism are often at greater risk of experiencing stress and lower quality of life, in comparison to parents of typically developing children and other developmental disabilities (D'Arcy et al,2023). Therefore, increasing the accessibility of the therapeutic activities to incorporate them into everyday tasks can be beneficial as parents are less likely to feel like it is something else to '*fit in*'.

Language differences

It can be a common misconception amongst staff in education settings that multilingualism can cause communication difficulties. This can result in both under and over diagnosis of language difficulties in multilingual populations. Therefore, another key role of an SLT is to support staff to be able to identify language difficulties versus language differences.

The RCSLT (n.d.a) advises that all languages spoken should be assessed to gain a full understanding of a client's communicative abilities. Working in a largely rural area can make in-person interpreter availability challenging. Where appropriate, it can be easier to arrange for an interpreter to join via video call. However, due to Adrianna's cognitive differences and possible neurodiversity this would not have been appropriate. Ensuring accessibility for multilingual clients also extends to the reports, signposting and resources provided after assessment. This has been supported by advances in technology which have significantly improved access to translation tools and resources. For example, many NHS Trust websites now feature integrated translation functions, which help to make services more accessible to diverse populations.

Despite ongoing developments in the field, there continues to be a lack of standardised assessments for multilingual children. To address this, I prepared informal resources and incorporated elements of dynamic assessment to explore Adrianna's communication difficulties.

Best practice recommends meeting with the interpreter in advance of the session to brief them on its purpose and the materials to be used. This preparatory step is especially important when using informal assessment techniques, as it ensures the interpreter understands the type of information they need to gather and how it should be recorded for subsequent analysis.

Approaches to delivering Speech and Language Therapy

Approach: Consultative approaches

Although it was not an issue in this case, a common barrier in my role can be supporting parents and caregivers to understand the consultative model of Speech and Language Therapy . Some may assume that it is solely the SLT's responsibility to work directly with the child on their targets. However, this is often not the case. The best outcomes, particularly in terms of generalisation, are achieved when a child's targets are supported consistently across different contexts.

Due to the constraints of our service model, it was not possible to provide direct intervention with Adrianna. However, her setting is highly proactive in supporting children with speech, language, and communication needs (SLCN). I was therefore confident at the point of discharge that staff would continue to work with her directly and support her ongoing progress. I meet termly with the school's in-house communication team and Special Educational Needs Coordinator (SENCo) to discuss the setting's SLCN provision, including ongoing therapy, new referrals, and children requiring review assessments after achieving their targets. This model enables me to indirectly monitor Adrianna's progress and ongoing needs.

Questions for reflection and discussion

1. What might it be like for a parent/caregiver to hear that their child is neurodiverse?
2. What might it be like for a therapist to discuss a child's neurodiversity with their parent or caregiver?
3. What communication skills might be needed to have a discussion of this nature?
4. How can communication barriers affect relationships between professionals and clients, and what strategies can help overcome them?
5. In what ways can cultural and linguistic diversity influence people's experiences and perceptions of healthcare?
6. How can professionals remain aware of their own assumptions and biases, and why is this important for ethical practice?

Further reading

Autism and Bilingualism, 'Should autistic children learn more than one language':

https://autism-bilingualism.com/

Speech and Language UK, 'Children learning more than one language':

https://speechandlanguage.org.uk/educators-and-professionals/resource-library-for-educators/children-learning-more-than-one-language/

Speech and Language UK, 'Myth-busting: Bilingualism / English as an additional language':

https://speechandlanguage.org.uk/about-us/news-and-blogs/myth-busting-bilingualism-english-as-an-additional-language/

Meir, N., & Hindi, I. (2025). Different paths to multilingualism in Autism Spectrum Disorder (ASD): Naturalistic and non-interactive. ***Journal of Child Language.*** Cambridge University Press.

www.cambridge.org/core/journals/journal-of-child-language/article/different-paths-to-multilingualism-in-autism-spectrum-disorder-asd-naturalistic-and-noninteractive/312FD9C9516E8EDE639F8BC548A34946

Baumeister, F., Wolfer, P., & Solaimani, E. (2025). On the impact of exposure to different languages on Theory of Mind in neurotypical and autistic children. ***Bilingualism: Language and Cognition.*** Cambridge University Press.

www.cambridge.org/core/journals/bilingualism-language-and-cognition/article/on-the-impact-of-exposure-to-different-languages-on-theory-of-mind-in-neurotypical-and-autistic-children/9EB3F9AF70156ACDBC677021B4E63855

Pert, S. (2022). ***Working with Children Experiencing Speech and Language Disorders in a Bilingual Context.*** Routledge.

Further information

Theories

Blank Levels: a framework of questions designed by Marion Blank (Blank, Rose & Berlin, 1978). It consists of 4 levels of increasingly complex and abstract questions.

DSM-5 (Diagnostic and Statistical Manual of Mental Disorders (5th edition) is used as a standard classification for mental health professionals (American Psychiatric Association, 2022).

Functional communication is being able to communicate your wants and needs either verbally or using other non-verbal methods, e.g. pointing.

Imaginative play: a type of play where children use their imagination to create play scenarios beyond the concrete environment, for example storytelling, role-playing.

Approaches

Box Time is an intervention designed to support attention, listening and expressive language through structured adult-led group activities based on Attention Autism (Watson, Davies, & Winterton, 2017).

Consultative approaches are where therapists work indirectly by upskilling others to work with clients towards their targets in everyday environments.

EHCP is a legal document in England that outlines the support required by a child/young person with special educational needs to enable them to achieve their developmental and educational goals.

Informal assessment: the child's communication skills are evaluated play-based activities, observation, and conversation.

NDS: diagnostic multi-disciplinary team usually consisting of Speech and Language Therapists, Paediatricians, and Clinical Psychologists that assess children for neurodiversity.

Observation: informal assessment method that involves watching and listening to a client in a naturalistic or structured setting to gain information about their communication skills.

WellComm assessment is a screening tool that uses a traffic light system to rate communication abilities – red indicating the need for SLT assessment, amber indicating the need for targeted support in school, and green indicating age-appropriate skills

Values

Accessibility: any intervention must meet the needs of the individual. In this case, assessments conducted solely in English are often ineffective and may lead to poorer outcomes and potential language attrition for multilingual children (RCSLT, 2023). Failing to provide an appropriate interpreter constitutes a form of discrimination under the Equality Act (UK Government, 2010).

Neuroaffirming practice: an inclusive, strengths-based approach that looks to support neurodiverse individuals through acknowledging and supporting their individual differences.

References

American Psychiatric Association. (2022). ***DSM-5-TR: Diagnostic and Statistical Manual of Mental Disorders*** (5th Ed). American Psychiatric Association

Blank, M., Rose, S. A. & Berlin, L. J. (1978). ***The Language of Learning: The Preschool Years***. Grune & Stratton, Inc.

D'Arcy, E., Burnett, T., Capstick, E., Elder, C., Slee, O., Girdler, S., Scott, M., & Milbourn, B. (2023). The well-being and support needs of Australian caregivers of neurodiverse children. ***Journal of Autism and Developmental Disorders, 54***(5). https://doi.org/10.1007/s10803-023-05910-1

Inan, S., & Harris, Y. R. (2025). Beyond the home: Rethinking heritage language maintenance as a collective responsibility. ***Frontiers in Psychology, 16***, 1616510. https://doi.org/10.3389/fpsyg.2025.1616510

RCSLT. (n.d.a). ***Bilingualism – Clinical Information for SLTs.*** www.rcslt.org/speech-and-language-therapy/clinical-information/bilingualism/

RCSLT. (n.d.b). ***Autism – Guidance.*** www.rcslt.org/members/clinical-guidance/autism/autism-guidance/#section-4

RCSLT. (2023). ***Working with Interpreters.*** www.rcslt.org/members/clinical-guidance/childrens-services/childrens-services-guidance/working-with-interpreters/

UK Government. (2010). ***Equality Act 2010 (c. 15).*** The Stationery Office. www.legislation.gov.uk/ukpga/2010/15/contents

Watson, J., Davies, G., & Winterton, A. (2017). An evaluation of the Attention Autism approach with young children with autism. ***Good Practice Autism, 18***(2), 79–93.

Case study 7
Rosie: 'how can I help?'

Lauren Flannery

Case overview

Theory: Stroke

Theory: Cerebral palsy

Theory: Global developmental delay

Theory: Typical development

Rosie is a three-year-old girl referred to speech and language therapy due to concerns about delayed speech and language development. There were no major pregnancy or delivery difficulties, and she was born at term. However, shortly after birth, Rosie suffered a stroke. She subsequently received a diagnosis of cerebral palsy. Rosie presents with global developmental delay, particularly in expressive and receptive language (expressive language is the ability to use words, sentences, and gestures to express thoughts and ideas, whilst receptive is the ability to understand and process language). Rosie's language is not developing in line with the typical level expected for children of her age. She has recently started to vocalise more frequently and is beginning to use early communicative behaviours such as pointing, protesting, and making simple requests. Her understanding of language is developing, but she demonstrates difficulty following longer instructions and maintaining attention.

Rosie attends a private nursery for two days a week. Nursery staff have raised concerns about her communication, noting inconsistent responses to verbal prompts and limited use of spoken words. They also report challenges around her attention span, frequent emotional outbursts, and difficulty transitioning between activities. The nursery has asked for advice on how best to support her emerging communication, alongside behavioural strategies.

Meeting Rosie and her mum

Soon after referral, I visit the family at home to assess Rosie's communication needs in the home environment. I chat to Rosie's mum, Fiona, whilst Rosie plays nearby.

DOI: 10.4324/9781003668756-10

'Hello Fiona, thank you for having me today', I begin by saying. *'I know things can feel busy and overwhelming, so I really appreciate you taking the time to meet and tell me more about Rosie's current communication needs'.*

Fiona sighs and says, *'It's fine. Honestly, I didn't know what to expect. I'm just... I'm tired. All the time. It's a lot'.*

'It sounds like things have been really hard lately. Can you tell me a bit about how things have been at home with Rosie?' I ask.

Approach: Active listening

Fiona's voice wavers. *'She's... she's lovely. But it's like, this isn't the little girl I thought I was going to have. I feel terrible even saying that'.*

'It's okay', I say, reassuringly, *'It's brave of you to say it. So many parents feel grief for the version of parenthood they imagined, and that doesn't take away from how much you love her'.*

Value: Respect

'Some days I just don't know what I'm doing', says Fiona, *'My eldest, he's being assessed for oppositional defiant disorder. The six-year-old copies everything he does. And then there's Rosie, and I just... I can't split myself three ways. My husband's away most of the time for work. It's all on me'.* She looks somewhat despondent.

'That's an awful lot to be carrying on your own. How are you doing, really?' I gently enquire.

'Honestly? Not great. I've had depression on and off for years. Anxiety too. But this, this is something else. Some days I feel like I'm barely keeping us all afloat', says Fiona.

I receive this by replying, *'Thank you for being so open with me. I can see how much you're trying to keep everything together. My role here is to support Rosie's communication, but I also want to make sure you feel supported too. You're not alone in this'.*

Value: Reassurance

Fiona nods, *'I just want to be a good mum. I do. I want to help her. I just don't know how'.*

'And you are helping', I say, *'by asking for support. That's a huge step. We can take this one step at a time, together. We'll look at what's working, what's hard, and what might help – not just for Rosie, but for you too'.*

Approach: Strength-based

During my home visit I notice that although the home environment is physically safe and well-kept, there is a high emotional burden within the family system. Fiona describes feeling isolated and unsupported, particularly when her husband is away. She expresses guilt and helplessness, unsure how to connect with Rosie or respond to her behaviours. I observe minimal verbal interaction between mother and child, with Rosie often being left to play alone or with an electronic device.

Fiona says, *'I just want to be a better mum. I really do. But I don't always know what that looks like'.*

I respond, *'Just from sitting with you today, I can see how much you care. That wish to be a better mum? That's love. That's connection. It's already here'.*

Value: Empathy

'I hope so. I just don't want to get it wrong. Sometimes I leave her with the tablet just so I can think straight. I know it's not great, but it's the only time it's quiet', Fiona adds.

'That's completely understandable. We all need a moment to breathe. Maybe we can look together at some small ways to build connection in the everyday stuff – without making things feel even heavier?' I reply.

Fiona nods, *'I think I'd like that. I just don't know where to start'.*

'We'll start together. And we'll keep things realistic – no pressure, no judgment. Just support, at your pace', I say.

Value: Compassion

While Rosie is not experiencing overt abuse or harm, the cumulative risk posed by unmet emotional needs and caregiver stress is evident. I utilise parental interviews and rating scales to better understand parental perceptions of Rosie's speech, language, and communication needs (SLCNs) and assess their level of concern and general stress.

I identify safeguarding concerns related to parental coping capacity and emotional availability, which necessitate sensitive inter-professional collaboration. Recognising these risks was crucial to framing Rosie's needs, not only as a developmental delay, but as part of a broader context of vulnerability.

Approach: Inter-professional collaboration

Gathering further information at nursery

Following my home visit, I go to the nursery and speak to the teacher (Janet) who shares important insights into Rosie's behaviour and communication challenges in the nursery environment.

'We're doing our best with Rosie', explains Janet, *'but... some days are just really hard. Sometimes she gets so frustrated she'll throw things or push the other children. It can feel like it comes out of nowhere'.*

'That sounds challenging, for her, and for you all', I say.

Janet responds, *'It is. I don't think she's trying to be unkind. It's more like... she just can't cope. Like something's bubbling over inside and she doesn't know how to let it out'.*

'That makes a lot of sense. Behaviour like that can often be a child's way of telling us something – especially when they don't yet have the words to explain how they feel', I suggest.

Approach: Guiding

'Exactly. The tricky part is, we're not really sure what the message is. We've been asking ourselves: is it her attention? Or maybe her understanding? Or both? It's so hard to tell in the moment,' Janet says.

I reply, *'I really appreciate your honesty and it's okay not to have all the answers right now. Rosie's signals are subtle, and in a busy nursery, it's not always easy to slow down and figure them out but you've already noticed a pattern – that her frustration links to communication'.*

Value: Empowerment

I observe Rosie during unstructured play and structured activities, both at home and in the nursery. These observations highlight delayed expressive and receptive language, with strengths in non-verbal communication such as gesturing, face watching, mutual eye gaze, and turn-taking. Rosie's attention and listening skills appear variable, affected by environmental distractions and emotional state.

I observe that although her motor function was relatively preserved, Rosie presents with mild dyspraxia and dysarthria, affecting her speech coordination.

Theory: Dyspraxia

Theory: Dysarthria

Planning interventions for Rosie

Given Rosie's complex needs and her family's vulnerabilities, I develop a flexible intervention that balances communication goals with emotional safety. Instead of an intensive, parent-led programme, I prioritise therapeutic scaffolding, focusing on relational capacity and consistent adult responsiveness across settings. Small, achievable strategies like sharing picture books daily and celebrating communication attempts with reflective commentary help keep intervention meaningful and manageable, allowing Rosie's mother to feel capable and engaged rather than overwhelmed.

Theory: Emotional safety

Approach: Scaffolding

Theory: Relational capacity

The intervention combines direct therapy and indirect therapy input via parent coaching and nursery staff training. Recognising the strained caregiving context, I focus on Rosie's communication and on increasing mum Fiona's emotional availability and confidence. While structured therapy tasks aren't feasible for Fiona right now, she welcomes gentle encouragement and guidance. The emphasis is on enhancing parent–child interaction and supporting Rosie's communicative intent rather than focusing on speech production.

Approach: Intervention types

Theory: Parent–child interaction

I use in-the-moment coaching and video feedback, drawing on video interaction guidance, highlighting Fiona's strengths, such as responding to Rosie's gestures or sharing smiles. I model simple strategies like following Rosie's lead in play. We discuss emotional regulation informally, helping Fiona to pause and reflect before reacting.

Approach: Video interaction guidance

Theory: Emotional regulation

Knowing Rosie's home is a high-stress environment, I collaborate closely with nursery staff to optimise her learning context. Together, we introduce visual supports at snack time, simplified language, and increased wait times. The

Approach: Visual supports

staff are proactive and receptive, and I encourage them to share small successes with Fiona to help build trust.

I support nursery staff to observe Rosie's interactions systematically, helping them to recognise moments of communicative intent – whether gestures, vocalisations, or behaviours. We explore how visual supports, simpler language, and wait-time adjustments can reduce frustration and boost engagement.

Working closely with others deepens my understanding of Rosie's daily life and enables a shared care plan across settings. I also model communication strategies for both parents and nursery staff, ensuring Rosie receives consistent, responsive support despite home challenges. For Rosie, progress depends as much on relationship quality as on communication skills.

Outcomes

Over six months, I saw steady, meaningful progress. Rosie began using a few consistent words with gestures, and her confidence in play interactions grew. More striking was the shift in her mother, and sessions moved from despair to cautious hope. Fiona became more present, more playful, and spoke of feeling 'more connected' to Rosie, celebrating moments like hearing her say 'up' or book sharing.

The nursery staff noticed improved attention and engagement, especially one-to-one, and felt more confident in supporting Rosie's communication. Joint working also strengthened the relationship with Rosie's family. I measured progress not just in words gained, but in emotional connection, reduced stress, and growing trust across systems.

While Rosie continues to present with significant communication needs, the case demonstrated that relational safety and responsive caregiving can be foundational therapeutic outcomes. Rather than relying solely on clinical benchmarks, I judge progress based on family engagement, parent–child connection, and reduced parental stress. These are critical foundations for long-term success.

Reflections

Rosie's development was shaped not only by her cerebral palsy, but by the emotional and environmental realities of her early life, including poor maternal mental health and reduced attunement. These factors likely compounded her communication needs beyond her neurological profile.

Yet the case also highlights how protective factors, nurturing interactions at nursery, small shifts in parental engagement, and consistent multi-agency input could foster resilience. A strengths-based approach helped me build on these moments to support relational and communicative growth.

I knew from the outset that a holistic, child- and family-centred assessment approach was essential. A standard assessment focusing solely on receptive and expressive language would not have captured the full picture of Rosie's communication needs. Instead, I adopted a multi-factorial assessment model to consider the complex interplay of physiological, developmental, environmental, and psychosocial factors influencing communication.

Approach: Family-centred

Approach: Multi-factorial assessment

Throughout the process, I was guided by the World Health Organization's International Classification of Functioning, Disability and Health (WHO-ICF) framework (WHO, 2001; Moran et al., 2020). This framework gave me a holistic view of Rosie, reinforcing the need to look beyond impairments and consider the full spectrum of Rosie's lived experience, helping me to plan meaningful, individualised support. I integrated observations from nursery staff, parent reports, and information from my observations and direct assessments. I also considered the impact of parental mental health history and family dynamics, to understand the systemic influences on Rosie's development.

Theory: WHO-ICF

Balancing the social and medical models in SLT practice

My approach was influenced by both the medical and social models of disability. The medical model helped identify Rosie's neurological and developmental impairments, supporting the use of clinical tools to profile speech and language delay. However, it was the social model that

Theory: Models of disability

provided the most useful lens for me to understand the barriers Rosie faced in participating in communication and play, particularly the environmental limitations imposed by her family context and caregiving dynamics.

By integrating both models, I was able to take a compassionate and realistic view of intervention, acknowledging Rosie's neurological differences while also seeking to reduce environmental barriers and increase her functional participation.

Rosie's needs could easily have been viewed solely through a medical lens, as a child with impairments to be treated. However, this perspective risked overlooking the broader relational and systemic barriers affecting her development. Drawing on the social model of disability helped me reframe Rosie's challenges within her broader context. Her difficulties were not solely rooted in her impairments but were shaped by emotional dynamics, caregiving patterns, and the presence (or absence) of inclusive, responsive environments. Recognising this allowed me to see her environment as both a barrier and a potential facilitator.

Clinical decision-making

Several pivotal decisions shaped my approach to Rosie's care. Safeguarding was a significant challenge. Although there was no immediate harm, her mother's emotional withdrawal and distress with comments like '*I didn't ask for this*' and '*I just can't cope anymore*' raised serious concerns about emotional neglect. I felt torn between my duty to protect Rosie and the need to build trust with her mother. I had to carefully judge when to escalate concerns without breaking trust. Escalating too early risked rupturing the fragile therapeutic relationship. I questioned how to act proportionately, in a way that safeguarded Rosie effectively.

Approach: Safeguarding

Recognising the complexity of Rosie's needs, I called an inter-professional meeting to share concerns. Through collaboration with the health visitor, nursery, and paediatrician, we ensured that medical, developmental, and social factors were considered alongside her communication

Approach: Early help

support. Through joint discussions, we aligned our understanding of Rosie's profile, coordinated interventions, and planned a referral to Early help, to build a consistent, supportive network around her both at nursery and home.

Setting goals for Rosie was also challenging. While her communication needed structured support, for example, key word modelling (a strategy where important words are clearly spoken and emphasised to support understanding) and visual aids, I had to consider her mother's limited capacity to deliver therapy at home. I knew that pushing too hard risked overwhelming her and causing disengagement. So, I chose a strengths-based, realistic approach, focusing on low-effort, high-impact strategies that fit Rosie's routines and her mother's current ability.

Professional role and emotional strain

This case also challenged my own well-being and professional identity. At times, I felt helpless, particularly when witnessing maternal distress and recognising Rosie's unmet needs. It highlighted the emotional strain speech and language therapists (SLTs) can face when working within complex family systems, where empathy, advocacy, and therapeutic boundaries often blur. Reflective practice allowed me to stay grounded, maintain curiosity, and listen without judgement, even amidst distressing disclosures. Rosie's case reinforced the need for strong support structures for clinicians working in emotionally complex settings.

Ethical practice in emotionally complex contexts

Working with Rosie placed me in ethically complex situations where the 'right' course of action was rarely straightforward. I had to balance building a therapeutic relationship with safeguarding responsibilities; support a parent while challenging emotional avoidance; and maintain hope amidst real adversity. These moments demanded emotional literacy, clinical judgement, and space for reflection. Clinical supervision and team dialogue were vital in navigating these tensions.

This case reminded me of the importance of compassionate safeguarding, approaching concerns not to blame, but to understand and address the barriers preventing caregivers from being fully present and responsive to their child. I was reminded of my professional duty to report concerns such as emotional neglect, to keep clear documentation and information-sharing protocols, and to raise issues respectfully and without judgement. Throughout, I worked to build trust with caregivers whilst holding Rosie's wellbeing at the centre of my practice.

Implications for SLT practice and training

Rosie's case highlighted several key implications for my practice as an SLT. Therapy doesn't happen in isolation; being effective required me to draw on skills beyond communication, including an understanding of family dynamics, trauma, attachment, and multi-agency working.

Goal setting had to be realistic and sensitive to context. In a family under stress, I learned to value not only language gains, but also shifts in emotional availability and relational connection. Sometimes, the most meaningful intervention was helping a parent feel safe, seen, and capable.

This work was emotionally complex. Clinical supervision was vital in helping me process the demands and stay grounded in ethical, compassionate care. It also sharpened my awareness of compassion fatigue, vicarious trauma, and the importance of cultural humility, recognising how values, grief, and acceptance shape each family's journey.

Rosie's case reminded me that my role as an SLT goes far beyond building language skills; it's about helping children feel seen, heard, and safe. For children at the intersection of disability and disadvantage, this means showing up as a clinician, advocate, and ally.

Speech and language needs rarely occur in isolation. They are shaped by a child's development, family dynamics, and context. In complex cases, I've learned the importance of a holistic, compassionate approach, one that balances clinical insight with ethical responsibility, safeguarding awareness, and collaboration.

Questions for reflection and discussion

1. How can speech and language therapists effectively balance their role in communication support with their responsibilities around safeguarding?
2. In cases where parents are experiencing mental health challenges or reduced caregiving capacity, how can SLTs set goals that are both meaningful and realistically achievable?
3. What should practitioners consider when the needs of the child and the needs of the parent appear to be in conflict?
4. In what ways can a strengths-based approach, focusing on the parent–child relationship, support and enhance communication development?
5. How can SLTs use collaborative, inter-professional approaches to ensure consistent support for children with complex needs across home and educational settings?
6. What role does reflective supervision play in helping SLTs manage the emotional and ethical challenges of working within high-stress family systems?

Further reading

Best Start in SLCN: Supporting Evidence: www.gov.uk/government/publications/best-start-in-speech-language-and-communication

Cerebral Palsy Research Network. Cerebral Palsy Types of Therapies: https://cprn.org/cerebral-palsy-types-of-therapies/

McCarthy, E., et al. (2022). Family-centered care in early intervention: A systematic review of processes, outcomes and influencing factors. ***Child: Care, Health and Development*, *48***(1), 1–15. reflehttps://doi.org/10.1111/cch.12901

Social and Medical Models of Disability: www.ombudsman.org.uk/sites/default/files/FDN-218144_Introduction_to_the_Social_and_Medical_Models_of_Disability.pdf

Video Interaction Guidance: www.videointeractionguidance.net/

Further information

Theories

Cerebral palsy is a condition that affects movement and muscle control due to damage to the brain, impacting motor coordination (the ability to control and coordinate body movements)

and speech production (the process of using muscles in the mouth to produce spoken language) (National Institute of Neurological Disorders and Stroke, n.d.).

Dysarthria: a speech disorder caused by weakness or poor control of the muscles used for speaking, often resulting in slurred or slow speech that can be hard to understand.

Dyspraxia: a neurological condition where a person has difficulty planning and coordinating physical movements, including speech or motor tasks.

Emotional regulation is the ability to recognise, manage, and respond to one's emotions in a flexible and socially appropriate way, supporting well-being, communication, and relationships.

Emotional safety involves creating an environment where individuals and families feel secure, respected, and free from judgement or distress, enabling them to share openly, process difficult emotions, and engage meaningfully in care.

Global developmental delay is the term used when a child takes longer to reach certain development milestones, e.g., movement, speech, learning, and social skills, than other children of the same age (Antolovich & Cooper, 2024).

Models of disability: the **medical model** views disability as a problem located within the individual, caused by a medical condition or impairment, and focuses on diagnosis, treatment, and cure. Whereas the **social model** views disability as the result of societal and environmental barriers, rather than an individual's impairment, emphasising the need to remove obstacles to inclusion and participation (Robertson & Jaswal, 2024).

Parent–child interaction is the dynamic exchange of communication, behaviour, and emotional cues between a parent and child, which plays a crucial role in supporting the child's social, emotional, and language development.

Relational capacity: an individual's ability to form and sustain responsive, attuned, and emotionally supportive relationships, which are essential for communication development and well-being.

Stroke: temporary loss of blood flow to the brain that can cause damage to neurological structures.

Typical development refers to stages of physical, cognitive, and emotional development. By age three, children typically understand simple instructions, use three- to four-word sentences, possess a vocabulary of several hundred words, and are understood by familiar adults most of the time.

WHO-ICF: a framework to assess how a health condition affects a person's body functions, daily activities, and participation in society, considering both personal and environmental factors.

Approaches

Active listening: giving your full attention, noticing both verbal and non-verbal cues, and responding thoughtfully to show understanding, build trust, and ensure concerns are truly heard.

Early help: a preventative form of support that aims to provide timely, targeted assistance to children and families experiencing emerging difficulties, to improve outcomes and reduce the need for more intensive interventions later (Lucas & Archard, 2021).

Family-centred: recognising the central role of the family in a child's life and working in partnership with them to tailor care, support, and decision-making to their unique strengths, values, and needs.

Guiding: involves the therapist supporting and coaching others, such as parents or practitioners, through collaborative reflection and modelling, to build their confidence and skills in fostering a child's communication and development.

Inter-professional collaboration involves close working between professionals from different disciplines who share expertise, responsibility, and decision-making to provide holistic, coordinated support for individuals and families.

Intervention types: speech and language therapy largely consists of direct therapy (working on specific skills and behaviours with an individual) and indirect therapy (that involves supporting others to implement strategies and create environments that facilitate the individual's communication).

Multi-factorial assessment: a comprehensive approach that considers a range of physiological, developmental, environmental, and psychosocial factors to understand an individual's strengths, needs, and context in depth.

Safeguarding: proactively identifying and responding to risks of harm, abuse, or neglect, ensuring the safety, rights, and well-being of children and vulnerable individuals are protected through appropriate action and inter-professional collaboration (Royal College of Speech and Language Therapists [RCSLT], n.d.).

Scaffolding: involves offering structured, responsive support that builds on their existing knowledge or confidence, gradually reducing guidance as they develop greater independence and capability in a particular area.

Strength-based: focuses on identifying, building, and utilising an individual's existing skills, resources, and positive attributes to promote growth, resilience, and meaningful outcomes.

Video interaction guidance: is an evidence-based intervention that uses short video clips of positive interactions to help individuals reflect on and strengthen communication, relationships, and attunement with others (Dodsworth, Kelly, & Bond, 2021).

Visual supports: Images, objects, or symbols to enhance understanding, predictability, and communication.

Values

Compassion: recognising and responding to the emotional and practical needs of individuals and families with empathy and kindness.

Empathy: to understand and share in the feelings and perspectives of individuals and families, using this understanding to inform compassionate, respectful, and person-centred care.

Empowerment: recognising others' expertise, whilst providing encouragement, guidance, and practical assistance.

Reassurance: involves responding sensitively and supportively when individuals or families disclose personal or distressing information.

Respect: recognising the inherent dignity, values, and choices of individuals and families, and ensuring their voices are heard and honoured in all aspects of care and decision-making.

References

Antolovich, G., & Cooper, M. S. (2024). Global developmental delay: A global misnomer. ***Journal of Paediatrics and Child Health***, ***61***(1), 127. https://doi.org/10.1111/jpc.16701

Dodsworth, E., Kelly, C., & Bond, C. (2021). Video interaction guidance with families: A systematic review of the research. ***Educational and Child Psychology***, ***38***(3), 48–61. https://doi.org/10.53841/bpsecp.2021.38.3.48

Lucas, S., & Archard, P. (2021). Early help and children's services: Exploring provision and practice across English local authorities. ***Journal of Children's Services***, ***16***(1), 74–86. https://doi.org/10.1108/JCS-03-2020-0006

Moran, M., Bickford, J., Barradell, S., & Scholten, I. (2020). Embedding the International Classification of Functioning, Disability and Health in health professions curricula to enable interprofessional education and collaborative practice. ***Journal of Medical Education and Curricular Development***, *7*, 1–8. https://doi.org/10.1177/2382120520933855

National Institute of Neurological Disorders and Stroke. (n.d.). ***Cerebral Palsy***. U.S. Department of Health and Human Services. www.ninds.nih.gov/health-information/disorders/cerebral-palsy

Robertson, Z., & Jaswal, V. (2024). Barriers to inclusion: Incorporating the social model in the study of children's understanding of disability. ***Cognitive Development***, ***70***, 101435. https://doi.org/10.1016/j.cogdev.2024.101435

Royal College of Speech and Language Therapists (RCSLT). (n.d.). ***Duty of Care Guidance***. www.rcslt.org/members/delivering-quality-services/duty-of-care-guidance/

World Health Organization (WHO). (2001). ***International Classification of Functioning, Disability and Health: ICF***. https://iris.who.int/bitstream/handle/10665/42407/9241545429.pdf?sequence=1

Case study 8
Kevin: breaking barriers: reducing stigma and fostering inclusion

Jing Feng and Shin Ying Chu

Background and referral

Kevin is a 6-year-old boy with moderate autism spectrum disorder (ASD) who lives with his parents and three siblings. His mother left her job to become a full-time caregiver. He was referred for speech-language therapy at the age of 3 years because of speech delays. Although Kevin has made progress after three years of therapy, his mother remains visibly stressed. Kevin's behaviors, such as hand flapping, shouting, and tantrums, limit the family's social life and cause anxiety about public perception, leading to rare outings. A recent shopping mall incident in which Kevin's screaming embarrassed his siblings deepened their social withdrawal. Moreover, the mother struggles to balance caregiving with the needs of her other children, and her shift from a professional career to full-time care has affected her identity and social ties. I begin working with Kevin after his recent relocation, as he starts receiving weekly interventions under my clinical supervision.

Theory: Autism spectrum disorders

Assessment findings

Before starting weekly clinical interventions with Kevin, I aim to get a clear picture of his background and current needs. I begin by reviewing his medical records and speaking with his mother, who assists me in completing his medical history collection. I learn that Kevin was diagnosed with moderate ASD at the age of 3 at Kuala Lumpur General Hospital. He currently receives speech therapy, which helps him make some progress, but his development remains slow, and he still requires significant one-to-one support.

Approach: Case history taking

Theory: Heterogeneity

As a speech-language therapist (SLT), I know that children with ASD are marked by heterogeneity. To plan the therapy that truly suits Kevin, I need more detailed information.

DOI: 10.4324/9781003668756-11

Approach: Clinical observations and interviews

Together with the multidisciplinary team, I conduct clinical observations and structured interviews with Kevin and his mother. I want to understand his behaviour, communication, and family situation. During our observations, we focus on how Kevin uses language, his social interactions, play skills, behaviours, and interests. Our findings match his earlier diagnosis of moderate ASD.

During my interview with Kevin's mother, her answers support what we have observed. When I take Kevin's developmental history, I learn that he has delays in both language and social skills. Before he turned 2, he could say simple words like 'dad' and 'mum,' but then his language stopped progressing.

Through our conversations, it also becomes clear that Kevin's ASD has created many challenges for the family.

Kevin's mother shares, '*...We almost never go out as a family anymore. Last week at the mall, Kevin suddenly started screaming because the lights were too bright, and everyone just stared at us. My oldest son pulled his hands away from me and ran off. Later, he cried and said he never wanted to go out with us again. Now, the other two don't want to go anywhere. They even ask me, "Why does our brother always have to embarrass us?"*'

I respond, '*That sounds really tough. It must be heartbreaking trying to look after Kevin and also help your other kids feel okay.*'

Value: Empathy

She paused and said, '*I don't even know how to describe it. Since I quit my job to stay home, I feel like I'm spinning all day, doing therapy with Kevin, driving the other kids around, cooking, cleaning... Even when I'm trying to sleep, I'm thinking about how to handle his meltdowns tomorrow. Sometimes I feel like I'm not even "me" anymore, just a machine taking care of kids.*'

Theory: Holistic care

I tell her, '*I can hear how exhausted and stretched thin you're feeling. You're carrying so much on your shoulders. Would it be all right if we talked about some ways you could have even small moments for yourself? Little breaks might help you feel a bit more like yourself again.*'

She nods, and through these conversations, I start to see how the family is facing stress from many directions: not just from caring for Kevin's daily needs, but also from trying to meet the emotional needs of the other children, keeping up social relationships, and dealing with limited support. Kevin's mother also speaks about feeling stigma and worrying about how others look at their family. All of this made me realise that working with Kevin also means supporting his family's well-being.

Theory: Stigma

The results from the structured assessments match what we see during the observations and interviews. When I test his language skills using the scales, he scores below the average range for his age.

Approach: Structured assessment

Intervention design

Based on Kevin's speech-language and behavioural challenges, as well as the difficulties faced by his family, I held a team discussion involving myself, a special education teacher, and a counsellor. With guidance from my clinical supervisor, we decided to use a Family-Centred Model (FCM) as the main framework for Kevin's intervention. Together, we create a personalised plan that addresses both Kevin's needs and his family's context.

Approach: Multidisciplinary team

Approach: Clinical supervision

Theory: Family-Centred Model (FCM)

This plan focuses on supporting Kevin's expressive and receptive communication. We know that real progress will only happen if the home environment also supports his growth. So, I work closely with Kevin's mother and siblings to build a language-rich setting at home. In addition, one of the plan's goals is to reduce the internalised stigma within the family, so we offer psychoeducation sessions to help Kevin's mother and siblings better understand autism and what it means for Kevin. His siblings are invited to join the weekly therapy sessions and participate in shared activities.

Theory: Psychoeducation

We hope that by involving the whole family, we can not only support Kevin's development but also improve family relationships, reduce isolation, and build long-term resilience. With the mother's consent, the plan is implemented and adjusted as needed through regular team reviews. We

Value: Consent

monitor the outcomes using both structured feedback and informal reports from the family.

Initial outcomes

After two months of intervention, I wanted to get a sense of how things were going, so I sit down with Kevin's mother for a follow-up conversation. She shared that Kevin has made real progress in both communication and behaviour. One of the biggest changes is how he can now use the Picture Exchange Communication System (PECS).

Approach: Picture Exchange Communication System (PECS)

'At the beginning,' she says, *'he couldn't even hand me a picture card unless I prompted him. But now, just six weeks in, he goes and gets his folder on his own. There was this one time when things got really loud, and instead of melting down, he just grabbed my hand and pointed. I asked him, "Do you want to go home?" and he said, "Home." That's one of his PECS words. I was amazed.'*

'That's wonderful,' I say. *'Has it helped with his outbursts too?'*

'Very much. He's not screaming like before, and the head-banging has really gone down. I think just being able to tell us what he wants helps him stay calmer.'

I nod. *'And how about outings?'*

She smiles. *'Honestly, I didn't have much hope at first... but things have really changed. Like this Saturday, we went to the park together as a family for the first time. We only stayed for about 30 minutes, but Kevin played on the swings with his noise-cancelling headphones. He just hummed quietly, no screaming like before. And my oldest even held his hand and said, "Little brother's doing so well today." That meant a lot.'*

'That's such a beautiful moment.' I say. *'It really sounds like those small steps are adding up.'*

Approach: ABC charts

Approach: Visual schedules

'Yeah, we've also started using ABC charts and visual schedules at home. I thought it would be too much at first, but it's

helped a lot. Kevin feels more settled when he knows what's coming next.'

'That shows real growth,' I say, *'not just in his words, but in how he's managing emotions and transitions.'*

'We've even laminated symbol cards and placed them all over the house, like in the kitchen and bathroom. And his siblings are really getting into it. We made up this game called "PECS Treasure Hunt." It makes things fun and keeps everyone involved.'

Value: Positive reinforcement

'His meltdowns have dropped a lot, and even when they happen, they don't last as long, maybe 6 or 7 minutes now instead of 15. I feel like I actually understand him better. And as a family, we're finally starting to work more as a team.'

She pauses for a moment, then adds:

'Respite care has honestly been a lifesaver. Yesterday, while a volunteer took Kevin out for sensory play, I slipped away to a café for half an hour and had a hot chocolate... and for the first time in three years, I felt like I could breathe. It was just 30 minutes, but in that moment, it felt like the world had colour again. Before that, everything just felt... grey.'

'I'm so glad you had that moment for yourself.' I say. *'Even small breaks matter. It's okay to take time to recharge.'*

She nods slowly.

'I'll try. At least now... at least now I feel like trying actually means something.'

I look at her and say, *'It does. And remember, you're not doing this alone. We'll keep working together, step by step, to support Kevin, and to support you too.'*

Value: Partnership

Reflections

Kevin's case taught me that supporting a child with ASD means understanding both communication challenges and family dynamics. As an SLT, I saw how PECS not only improved Kevin's ability to express himself but also helped reduce his emotional outbursts. Communication, I realised, is not just about words; it's about helping children feel understood and regulated.

A key part of Kevin's progress came from his family's involvement. His mother and siblings actively took part in his therapy, which reinforced for me the importance of the FCM. However, I also realised that real family involvement means more than just following strategies; it requires emotional understanding. Kevin's mother was under significant stress, trying to care for him while also meeting the needs of her other children. This taught me that my role as an SLT is not only to provide tools, but also to listen and offer support with empathy. Rather than assigning rigid tasks, I collaborated with her to find simple, natural ways to build communication into daily routines without adding to her burden. At first, Kevin's siblings were reluctant to join therapy. Through games and storytelling, they slowly became more understanding and supportive. This shift helped strengthen family bonds, which are essential for long-term success.

Theory: Neurodiversity

Approach: Speech-language therapist (SLT) role

This case reminded me that therapy doesn't end in the clinic. Family stress, inconsistent routines, and social stigma all impact progress. I saw that effective support must be flexible, patient, and ongoing. More broadly, Kevin's journey prompted me to reflect on neurodiversity and how society perceives autism. Inclusion is not just about accepting differences, it requires meaningful action. As SLTs, our role goes beyond the therapy room; we must also act as advocates, promoting care that is compassionate, fair, and culturally responsive.

Questions for reflection and discussion

1. Why is it important to think about both the child's behaviour and the family's well-being when planning interventions?
2. What might cause families of children with ASD to feel isolated?
3. How can we support families without making them feel like they must handle everything on their own?

4. What can help different professionals work well together to support families in a family-centred way?
5. How can therapeutic interventions be designed to strengthen sibling relationships and promote family cohesion?
6. How can speech-language therapists balance the dual role of clinical expert and family advocate?

Further reading

Autismspeaks: www.autismspeaks.org/

Autistica: www.autistica.org.uk/

Botha, M., Dibb, B., & Frost, D. M. (2022). "Autism is me": An investigation of how autistic individuals make sense of autism and stigma. ***Disability & Society*, *37***(3), 427–453.

Kinnear, S. H., Link, B. G., Ballan, M. S., & Fischbach, R. L. (2016). Understanding the experience of stigma for parents of children with autism spectrum disorder and the role stigma plays in families' lives. ***Journal of Autism and Developmental Disorders*, *46***(3), 942–953.

National Autistic Society (NAS): www.autism.org.uk/

Further information

Theories

Autism spectrum disorders are brain-based conditions that affect communication, social interaction, and behaviour. Signs may include poor eye contact, strong routines, or sensitivity to sounds. Because each person is different, it is called a 'spectrum.' Diagnosis is based on DSM-5 criteria.

Family-Centred Model (FCM) values the family as an active partner in planning and delivering care. It focuses on the child's needs within the family context, respecting family strengths, choices, and everyday routines (Watling et al., 2023).

Heterogeneity means that autism looks different in every person. Some may have strong language skills, while others may not speak at all. Because of this, support must be tailored to each person's unique needs (Mottron & Bzdok, 2020).

Holistic care means helping the whole child, not just with their speech, but also their feelings, daily life, and family situation. SLTs look at all these areas to give better support.

Neurodiversity is the idea that differences in brain function like ASD are natural variations, not disorders to be fixed. It promotes acceptance, inclusion, and respect for all ways of thinking and learning (Gupta & Aman, 2025).

Psychoeducation means helping families learn about ASD so they can understand it better, feel less worried, and make more confident choices.

Stigma refers to the negative views or stereotypes that people may have about conditions like ASD. It can cause families to feel judged or isolated, and may stop them from getting help, making it harder to support the child (Salleh et al., 2020).

Approaches

ABC Charts are tools that track behaviour by noting what happened before (Antecedent), what the child did (Behaviour), and what happened after (Consequence) (Dyer, 2013). They help find patterns and plan better support.

Case history taking means gathering information about a child's development and communication by talking to parents and reviewing records. It helps professionals understand the child's needs and plan suitable support.

Clinical observations and interviews are ways to learn more about a child by watching how they behave and talking with their caregivers. This helps SLTs understand the child's needs in real-life situations and plan the right support.

Clinical supervision means that a more experienced professional guides and supports a less experienced one. It helps make sure practice is safe, thoughtful, and effective, especially in complex cases.

Multidisciplinary team means a group of professionals from different fields, like SLTs, teachers, and doctors, working together to support a child. In ASD, this teamwork helps create a well-rounded plan to meet the child's different needs (Strunk et al., 2017).

Picture Exchange Communication System (PECS) teaches children to use pictures to ask for things and make choices. It is often used with non-speaking or minimally verbal autistic children to help them communicate more independently (May et al., 2025).

Speech-language therapist (SLT) role goes beyond teaching speech. It includes assessing needs, supporting families, collaborating across settings, and advocating for inclusive, person-centred care.

Structured assessment uses standard tools to measure a child's communication, behaviour, or development in a consistent way. In Kevin's case, structured assessments supported but did not replace clinical observations. They provided extra data to confirm findings and guide planning.

Visual schedules use pictures to show what will happen next. They help autistic children feel more prepared, reduce stress, and become more independent in daily routines.

Values

Consent means asking for clear permission before starting therapy. SLTs explain what will happen, respect the person's choice, and make sure they feel safe and informed.

Empathy means understanding others' feelings and showing care. For SLTs, it means listening kindly, supporting families with patience, and building trust to help therapy work better.

Partnership means working together with families. It is about sharing decisions, respecting each other, and supporting the child as a team.

Positive reinforcement means rewarding good behaviour with praise or something the child or parents likes. It helps build confidence and encourages learning in therapy.

References

Dyer, K. (2013). Antecedent-behavior-consequence (ABC) analysis. In ***Encyclopedia of autism spectrum disorders*** (pp. 175–180). Springer, New York, NY.

Gupta, A., & Aman, N. (2025). Embracing neurodiversity: The critical role of awareness and acceptance in autism spectrum disorders. ***Archives of Molecular Biology and Genetics***, ***4***(1), 1–8.

May, R. J., Salman, H., O'Neill, S. J., Denne, L., Grindle, C., Cross, R., Roberts-Tyler, E., Meek, I., & Games, C. (2025). Exploring the use of the picture exchange communication system (PECS) in special education settings. ***Journal of Autism and Developmental Disorders***, 1–15.

Mottron, L., & Bzdok, D. (2020). Autism spectrum heterogeneity: Fact or artifact? ***Molecular Psychiatry***, ***25***(12), 3178–3185.

Salleh, N. S., Abdullah, K. L., Yoong, T. L., Jayanath, S., & Husain, M. (2020). Parents' experiences of affiliate stigma when caring for a child with autism spectrum disorder (ASD): A meta-synthesis of qualitative studies. ***Journal of Pediatric Nursing***, ***55***, 174–183.

Strunk, J., Leisen, M., & Schubert, C. (2017). Using a multidisciplinary approach with children diagnosed with autism spectrum disorder. ***Journal of Interprofessional Education & Practice***, ***8***, 60–68.

Watling, R., Benevides, T., & Robertson, S. M. (2023). Family-centered interventions for children on the autism spectrum (2013–2021). ***The American Journal of Occupational Therapy***, ***77***(Supplement 1), 7710393210.

Case study 9
Noah: working together to approach bullying and stuttering in childhood

Rachael Unicomb

Case background

Noah is a ten-year-old boy who currently attends primary school and lives at home with his mother, Joan, and his two younger siblings: Theo who is eight, and Isla who is four. Noah's parents divorced when he was five years old, and Joan reports the parental relationship is an amicable one, with both parents having joint custody of the children. Noah enjoys playing football, spending time with his friends, and going to school. His favourite subjects at school are maths and science, and Noah wants to study engineering at university one day.

Noah's father, Liam, has recently remarried. Joan has recently gotten a new job and has subsequently moved to live in a new suburb about 30 minutes from her previous residence. Noah's parents have decided to enrol the children into a new school closer to Joan's home. About two months after Noah started at his new school, both Joan and Liam noticed some changes in the way Noah communicates and interacts. Noah appeared to have a reduced interest in his schoolwork, even for his favourite subjects, and had started waking up saying he does not want to go to school. He was quieter than usual, not talking as much as he normally would. Noah has always been described as a sociable, confident, and cheerful boy by those who know him well. His friends and family also say he is very talkative, funny, and outgoing. Noah has a stutter.

Theory: Stuttering

Joan and Liam suspect Noah is being teased and/or bullied at his new school and have set up a meeting with Liam's teacher and school counsellor to discuss this. Noah recently approached his parents and asked them, *'Can I please go back to speech therapy again to help me with my speaking?'* Noah's parents were unable to get him an appointment with the speech-language therapist (SLT) who saw him as a young child, though have made

Theory: Bullying

DOI: 10.4324/9781003668756-12

an appointment at a new service with me. When I first meet Noah and his family, I have been working as an SLT in a private clinic for just under a year and have very little experience (outside of my university studies) working with children who stutter.

Gathering a case history

As part of my first meeting with Noah, I gather an extensive background/case history from him and his parents.

Approach: Gathering case history

I begin by asking his parents, '*When did you first notice Noah's stutter?*'

Value: Family-centred care

Joan replies, '*It was just before his fourth birthday*'.

'*It seemed to come on gradually*', she said, '*he mostly repeated sounds and words to begin with. It wasn't all that noticeable really. But it seemed to get worse when he was tired, excited, or trying to compete for talking time with his brother and sister.*'

'*Do you think there are times now when you seem to stutter more, Noah?*' I ask him.

He shrugs. His mum continues, '*When it first started, Noah was in preschool, and it didn't seem to bother him. I don't ever remember him being frustrated or upset by it. And his preschool teachers always said he was a happy and sociable boy there*'.

Value: Responsiveness and empathy

Noah's dad says that they took him to see his previous SLT just before he turned five, prior to starting formal schooling. There, he was diagnosed with stuttering. In collaboration with Noah's parents, treatment commenced immediately, utilizing a holistic approach (combining direct and indirect strategies/treatments) aiming to educate family members about stuttering, and facilitate increased fluency, effective communication, and a positive communicative environment. Noah's parents worked with that SLT for eight weeks; however, they were in the process of separating/divorcing, and implementing regular home therapy became difficult. It was mutually decided to cease therapy at that time due to the competing familial demands.

'We didn't go back to speech therapy after that', Noah's mum adds, *'everything seemed ok. Noah was fine – he loved school and engaged well in the classroom. Nobody else seemed to notice his stutter'*.

'And what's changed now?' I ask.

'Well' says his dad, *'he's just recently moved to a new primary school, and we've been a bit worried about him'*.

Assessing Noah

Noah had been previously diagnosed with stuttering, so assessment considerations were around determining the current extent and nature of Noah's stuttering and assessing any change over time (not only related to speech behaviours, but more significantly, related to the potential impact of the stuttering on Noah). I thoroughly assess Noah's stuttering and note it is predominantly characterized by repetitions (of incomplete-, complete-, and multisyllables), and fixed postures with and without audible airflow (i.e., sound prolongations and blocks). Noah shows some signs of frustration when he stutters. I also assess the impact of stuttering on Noah, using the Overall Assessment of the Speaker's Experience of Stuttering: School-age Children (OASES-S). Capturing Noah's own experiences during the assessment demonstrates valuing the child's voice in understanding the impact of stuttering. Noah's OASES-S results are summarized in Table 9.1 and indicate Noah's self-reported degree of adverse impact that stuttering has on his life as moderate.

Theory: Overall Assessment of the Speaker's Experience of Stuttering: School-age Children (OASES-S)

I talk through these results in more detail with Noah to find out more about his feelings and perceptions around his stuttering in his own words. I start out by asking him, *'Noah, do you think you can tell me what it feels like for you when you stutter?'*

He replies, *'It feels like my words get stuck in my throat and I can't get them out, and it's really embarrassing'*.

'That sounds like it would be very frustrating for you, Noah,' I respond. *'I'd really like to try and help you with your*

Assessment Section and Purpose	Impact Score	Impact Rating
I – General Information Assesses the child's knowledge of stuttering and how they feel about/their perception of their stuttering and general communication abilities.	3.38	Moderate–severe
II – Reactions to Stuttering Assesses the child's affective (emotional), behavioural, and cognitive reactions to their stuttering (e.g., frustration, embarrassment, avoidance behaviours, etc.).	3.25	Moderate–severe
III – Communication in Daily Situations Assesses how stuttering affects the child's communication in various everyday situations (e.g., in the classroom, with friends, etc.).	2.20	Mild–moderate
IV – Quality of Life Assesses the impact of stuttering on the child's overall quality of life (e.g., impact on social interactions, activities, and participation, etc.).	2.78	Moderate
OVERALL IMPACT SCORE	**2.93**	**Moderate**

Table 9.1 Summary of OASES-S assessment results for Noah

communication if I can. Can you tell me, how do you feel when you stutter at school, or at home, or with friends?'

Noah replies, *'I don't like to speak in class. Even if I know the answer, I won't put my hand up because I don't want people to laugh at me or think I'm weird. But I feel better when I'm talking with my friends, and my dog, and Mum and Dad'.*

Goal setting

Approach: Collaborative goal setting

Value: Psychosocial wellbeing and emotional safety

Using the findings from my assessment, I plan goals with Noah and his parents. At Noah's age, treatment goals for stuttering need to be holistic, multifaceted, and personalized. Goals may focus not only on reduction of disfluency (if that is important to Noah). They should consider Noah's overall communication experiences in all relevant environments, consider his activities and participation, and any impact on his quality of life. In that way, treatment goals may address the whole communication experience and may focus on the behavioural, cognitive, and/or affective aspects of the disorder. For Noah, this may involve focusing on communicative interactions in the classroom; facilitating positive social interactions; minimizing any situational or verbal avoidance behaviours; and increasing self-acceptance, and/or increased fluency.

I discuss treatment goals directly with Noah. He tells me, *'I want help with my talking. I don't want to stutter as much at school. I don't like stuttering there. I just don't want to be embarrassed anymore when Miss asks me a question in class.'*

'This is certainly something we can work on together', I say. Hearing this, he smiles for the first time in the session.

As I am wrapping up the goal-setting discussion, I ask him, *'Is there anything else I can help you with, or that you want me to know?'*

Noah's voice starts to quiver, and he puts his head down and quietly says to me and his parents, *'There is a kid at my new school, Beau, he's been really mean to me, teasing me, calling me names, and copying my stuttering. He makes all the other kids laugh at me.'*

I then gently ask him, *'Noah, how often does Beau do this to you at school?'*

Eyes welling up with tears, he replies, *'Every day. I just want kids to know that I'm smart and funny. I just get stuck sometimes'*.

Noah has just disclosed he is being bullied at school. Noah attributes this directly to his stuttering, and therefore one of his main goals was to reduce bullying and stigma, as well as working on communication.

Value: Advocacy and safeguarding

A collaborative approach to support Noah

Moving forward, I work closely with Noah, his family, and other professionals to support his communication and

Value: Teamwork

psychosocial goals. A collaborative, team-based approach is essential to ensure that all aspects of Noah's wellbeing – communication, emotional health, social development, and academic success – are being met. I will now outline my considerations around how each of these roles/people support Noah as part of a collaborative team.

My role

Theory: Aims of therapy

In relation to Noah's communication focused goals, the SLT role can aim to improve overall communication. This may, in turn, support increased self-confidence. I provide education to Noah and his parents/family around stuttering and working with other professionals to continue to advocate for support of Noah and his needs. Education to Noah's parents is also given around how they can support Noah and his communication and social goals at home, and at school. It is also important for me to monitor for signs of social anxiety and other psychosocial issues that may warrant referral and investigation to other professionals. Noah may need a referral to relevant mental health professionals around how he is feeling about himself and about the bullying that is happening to him, for example, to school counsellors and/or psychologists. I can also work with Noah's parents, teachers, mental health professionals, and peers to support building self-efficacy, increase self-esteem, provide strategies around reduction of negative listener responses, reduce bullying by educating peers and others about stuttering, and increase self-regulation and resilience.

Caregivers and families

Value: Open communication and emotional safety

Value: Autonomy and child voice

I provide advice to Noah's parents to support him at home. I advise that Noah's parents take time to listen to him and never talk over him or try to complete his sentences. They should not feel the need to avoid talking about stuttering with Noah or their other children. Noah's speech should never be mocked or imitated. These strategies will also be important for Noah's parents to model on their younger children, so the home is a supportive environment for him.

It will be important for Noah's parents and family to actively seek out his thoughts/feelings and opinions, and to be his advocate when he wants them to be. This will facilitate building Noah's self-confidence. To support Noah in relation to bullying, I advise his parents to be calm and positive with him at home. They have already set up a meeting with Noah's school, and this is a positive step. Noah's parents should encourage him to talk to them about what is happening, so they can provide him with appropriate strategies that he can manage himself at school for dealing with situations as they arise. As friendships are a protective factor for bullying, it will be important for Noah's parents to potentially facilitate positive peer interactions/experiences at his new school, but also to ensure that existing supportive friendships (e.g., at previous school, football team, etc.) are maintained.

Teachers and school staff

I provide advice and support to Noah's teachers. I encourage his teacher to ask Noah if he feels comfortable speaking aloud in front of the class, and if so, whether he would like to be called upon to do so in a certain order. Similarly, the teacher should also be using some of the communicative strategies that his parents are using at home (e.g., not speaking over the top of him or finishing his sentences, etc.). The teacher may also ask Noah whether they can talk to his classmates about stuttering to help them understand more about it. If Noah is amenable to this idea, the teacher can work with me (as his SLT) to obtain/access relevant child-friendly information about stuttering to present to the class.

Value: Respect and dignity

Value: Empathy and awareness

Approach: Raising awareness of bullying

Mental health professionals

Resilience is a factor that may not only protect people from the negative impacts of stuttering across the lifespan, but also the impacts of bullying. Mental health professionals will be able to assess Noah's overall mental health (being mindful of social anxiety and depression, etc.), and coping mechanisms, including resilience skills. There are a range of evidence-based programmes and strategies that can be delivered by relevant mental health professionals to support Noah in relation to building resilience. Further, they can assist with working on building self-efficacy/confidence, and support building positive social relationships. If Noah shows signs of social anxiety, they may provide cognitive restructuring or other relevant strategies/intervention as required. These professionals will also be able to assist with anti-bullying education and intervention.

Peers

Working with Noah's teacher, I advise on how his peers can play a crucial role in supporting his goals by helping to create an inclusive, understanding, and confidence-building environment. They can encourage inclusion by inviting him to actively participate in all conversations and help him feel like a valued group member. They may call out teasing and bullying if they see it happening to Noah. They can actively learn about stuttering to understand that it is a speech/communication difference, not a reflection of intelligence or ability, helping reduce stigma around the disorder.

Value: Belonging and shared experience

Finally, Noah may benefit from the support of other peers who stutter. I recommend that if Noah is agreeable to it, Noah's family should actively seek out support groups in their area for his age group, if available. Support groups help foster a feeling of being understood and accepted and may help Noah realize there are others who share similar experiences to him.

My role as SLT is essential in working with lots of individuals around Noah to provide supportive strategies to facilitate communication and psychosocial goals and support him in relation to bullying using interventions/strategies that are evidence-based, age- and culturally appropriate for Noah.

Reflections

As a recently qualified SLT, I found working with Noah both rewarding and challenging. I was struck by the complexity of his case – not just the clinical aspects of stuttering, but the emotional and social layers shaped by bullying, family transitions, and Noah's own self-perception. I felt a strong sense of responsibility to advocate for Noah while also navigating my limited experience in managing cases involving psychosocial impacts. Collaborating with Noah's family, school staff, and mental health professionals highlights the importance of teamwork and holistic care and reminds me that effective therapy goes beyond fluency management – it involves listening, empowering, and supporting the child in all aspects of their life. This case deepened my appreciation for child-centred practice and the value of interprofessional collaboration in achieving meaningful outcomes.

Clinical considerations of stuttering

Theory: Stuttering tractability

Approach: Holistic care

As children move from preschool-age to school-age, stuttering becomes less tractable, and the disorder is more likely to become persistent in nature. When a child reaches this age, they are spending more time at school, and less time with families. Children experience significant physical and emotional changes during this time as they navigate developmental, social, and educational demands. If a child is also stuttering, they may face additional pressures in some of these domains. Assessment of a child who stutters at this age needs to therefore be comprehensive and holistic. A clinician should gain a thorough understanding of how the child feels about their stuttering/communication in general and look closely for any signs of potential negative psychosocial impacts of stuttering on the child (American Speech-Language-Hearing Association (ASHA), n.d.).

Stuttering and wellbeing

Value: Mental health awareness and trauma-informed care

The literature highlights that stuttering may have a potential negative impact on the lives of some individuals. For a child who stutters, there can be educational and classroom-based challenges, social impact (e.g., social/situational avoidance, impact on peer/interpersonal relationships, etc.), impact on self-confidence/esteem, impact on self-perceived communicative competency and on overall quality of life. There is also potential for negative impact on mental health.

For children who stutter, evidence indicates that psychological issues, including social anxiety, may originate in the school years, with approximately one quarter of school-aged children who stutter diagnosed with social anxiety disorder.

Bullying can have a significant impact on the psychological wellbeing of any child, and the impacts of bullying can be serious, and long-reaching.

Theory: Impact of bullying

Bullying in childhood: red flags, risk and protective factors

There are various psychological and social theories/frameworks around why bullying may occur, that aim to highlight contributing factors for why a perpetrator may bully others (see Varlik, 2024, for a full summary around theories).

Noah's parents tell his teacher about Beau bullying Noah at school.

Theory: Self-esteem and social isolation theory of bullying

Noah's teacher tells them, '*Beau has had a difficult upbringing and childhood. He struggles with self-esteem and feels left out by other peers, so he seems to try to compensate for this in other ways with less desirable behaviour*'. Noah's teacher thinks that this could be a potential underlying reason why Beau is bullying Noah.

Bullying can result in very harmful implications without intervention. For caregivers/parents, educators, and professionals working with children, it is therefore essential to be aware of potential red flags for identification of bullying, as well as associated risk and protective factors to ensure early detection and timely support.

Bean (2008) summarizes potential indicators that a child may be being bullied, some of which include:

- Acting (uncharacteristically) aggressively and/or unreasonably.
- Change in sleep and eating patterns.
- Presenting with unexplained injuries.
- Change in academic performance.
- Being alone and/or excluded by peers.
- Missing or damaged personal effects.
- Frequent, unexplained tears and mood swings.
- Not wanting to go to school and/or seeking alternative methods for getting to school.
- Unexplained health conditions (headaches, stomach aches, etc.).
- Avoiding certain people and places.
- Talks about being verbally or physically teased and/or threatened.
- Talks about self-blame, reports general feelings of lack of self-worth.

Understanding and addressing risk and protective factors for bullying is also essential to development of targeted interventions that not only reduce the likelihood of bullying but also strengthen the child's support system and coping abilities. Johansson (2023) summarizes potential risk factors for children as victims of bullying to include: family factors (e.g., instability in home/family structure, negative parenting), personal factors (e.g., exposure to prior bullying, physical and/or psychological characteristics), school factors (e.g., lack of or limited: anti-bullying education/interventions, teacher support, and staff monitoring), and peer factors (e.g., isolation, exclusion, limited social acceptance/support). Protective factors are summarized similarly and relate to family factors (e.g., stable home/family life, positive parenting strategies involving open communication, trust, and support), personal factors (e.g., good academic performance and social skills, good sense of self), school factors (e.g., education and intervention programmes around bullying, supportive teacher–student relationships), and peer factors (e.g., having best friends and a group of mutual friends).

Value: Prevention and early intervention

Questions for reflection and discussion

1. In what ways do you think SLTs can support a child who stutters and is being bullied within the scope of our practice?
2. How might a SLT advocate for systemic change within schools to better support students who stutter and experience bullying?
3. How can SLTs use collaborative, interprofessional approaches to support a child who stutters and is being bullied?
4. Which theories regarding why bullying occurs do you think most lend themselves to why children who stutter might be bullied, and why?
5. What are the potential risks of overlooking the emotional and social dimensions of stuttering in school-aged children like Noah?
6. What do you think could be done at a wider, systematic level to educate the general public about stuttering?

Further reading

Blood, G. (2012). Bullying and SLPs: Enhancing our roles as advocates. ***The Stuttering Foundation.*** www.stutteringhelp.org/content/bullying-and-slps-enhancing-our-roles-advocates

Cozart, G., & Wilson, L. (2022). Strategies for teachers to support children who stutter: Perspectives of speech-language pathologists. ***Perspectives of the ASHA Special Interest Groups***, *7*, 73–86.

Johnson, G., Onslow, M., Horton, S., & Kefalianos, E. (2023). Psychosocial features of stuttering of stuttering for school-age children: A systematic review. ***International Journal of Language and Communication Disorders***, ***58***, 1829–1845. doi: 10.1111/1460-6984.12887

Lowe, R., Menzies, R., O'Brian, S., Onslow, M., & Packman, A. (2023). Supporting a student who stutters: What schools can do. ***Scan***, ***42***(1), 52–55.

Yaruss, S., Reeves, N., & Herring, C. (2018). How speech-language pathologists an minimize bullying of children who stutter. ***Seminars in Speech and Language***, ***39***(4), 342–355. doi: 10.1055/s-0038-1667163

Further information

Theories

Aims of therapy in stuttering intervention include increased fluency, communicating more easily/effectively, supporting social communication, increasing acceptance and self-advocacy about stuttering, and minimizing situational and communicative avoidance (Druker et al., 2019).

Bullying is deliberate, repetitive behaviour which causes physical, social, and/or emotional harm to someone who has (or is perceived to have) less power. A perpetrator of bullying will often target individuals who are vulnerable or unprotected, including individuals with a form of disability (Varlik, 2024).

Impact of bullying: bullying is linked with poor academic performance, difficulties transitioning through life stages (e.g., into adolescence, moving from primary to secondary schooling), and serious mental health concerns. Children with a disability (including those with communication-related issues) are more vulnerable to being bullied. Children who stutter are at an increased risk of being teased and bullied compared to their peers who do not stutter, which in turn elevates risk of social anxiety (Bernard et al., 2022).

Overall Assessment of the Speaker's Experience of Stuttering: School-age Children (OASES-S) is an assessment for children aged 7–12 years and aims to understand (from the child's own direct report) how stuttering affects their emotional wellbeing, communication, and overall quality of life (Yaruss et al., 2016).

Self-esteem and social isolation theory of bullying: states that a perpetrator may bully others to try and make themselves feel better, or protect their own self-esteem, as they may feel worthless or excluded.

Stuttering is a fluency-related communication disorder that impacts the forward-flow of an individual's speech. It is characterized by involuntary speech disruptions, such as repetitions, fixed articulatory postures (also known as prolongations and blocks), which are often accompanied by physical tension and secondary behaviours. Stuttering can impact on communicative effectiveness and psychosocial wellbeing due to both (negative) speaker and listener reactions.

Stuttering tractability means that stuttering appears to be less responsive to treatment as a person gets older. Stuttering is thought to be at its most responsive to treatment in early childhood (closer to stuttering onset) but becomes less responsive as the child grows older into adolescence and adulthood, as indicated by effect sizes found in results of clinical trials (Onslow, 2025).

Approaches

Collaborative goal setting ensures that treatment priorities are co-developed with the child and their caregivers, promoting shared ownership, relevance, and alignment with the child's personal communication needs and values.

Gathering case history: this is a clinical process whereby an SLT collects detailed information about a child's developmental, medical, familial, educational, and communicative background to inform assessment, diagnosis, and individualized treatment planning.

Holistic care: involves addressing not only speech fluency but also the emotional, social, and environmental factors that influence the child's overall communication and wellbeing.

Raising awareness of bullying: schools need to ensure that anti-bullying campaigns and interventions are utilized, based on raising awareness around bullying (what it is, what it looks like, what to do if you are being bullied, or see someone being bullied), sensitization, and empathy building (Varlik, 2024).

Values

Advocacy and safeguarding: recognizing and responding to bullying reflects the clinician's role as an advocate for the child's safety and psychological wellbeing.

Autonomy and child voice: supporting the child's choice in when and who to be advocated for respects their autonomy and values their voice.

Belonging and shared experience: peer support groups promote belonging and validate shared experiences, which are essential for emotional growth and confidence.

Empathy and awareness: educating peers fosters empathy and reduces stigma, contributing to a more inclusive and respectful school culture.

Family-centred care: gathering a detailed case history from both the child and their caregivers reflects a commitment to family-centred practice, which values the lived experiences and insights of families in shaping assessment and intervention.

Mental health awareness and trauma-informed care: acknowledging the mental health implications of stuttering and bullying supports trauma-informed practice and holistic care.

Open communication and emotional safety: encouraging open dialogue fosters emotional safety and supports the child's confidence and self-expression.

Prevention and early intervention: reflects a proactive, values-driven approach to care that prioritizes early identification and support to mitigate harm.

Psychosocial wellbeing and emotional safety: reflects a commitment to supporting the child's emotional wellbeing and social development, increasing self-efficacy, self-confidence, and self-regulation; and/or increased fluency (ASHA, n.d.).

Respect and dignity: giving the child agency in classroom participation respects their dignity and promotes a supportive learning environment.

Responsiveness and empathy: recognizing and adapting to family circumstances reflects a value-driven approach that prioritizes empathy, flexibility, and realistic goal setting in clinical care.

Teamwork: when supporting a child who stutters, teamwork involves coordinated, respectful collaboration among professionals, caregivers, educators, and peers to ensure the child's communication, emotional, and social needs are met holistically and effectively.

References

American Speech-Language-Hearing Association (ASHA). (n.d.). ***Stuttering, cluttering, and fluency.*** www.asha.org/practice-portal/clinical-topics/fluency-disorders

Bean, A. L. (2008). ***Protect your child from bullying: Expert advice to help you recognize, prevent and stop bullying before your child gets hurts.*** Jossey-Bass.

Bernard, R., Hofslundsengen, H., & Frazier Norbury, C., (2022). Anxiety and depression symptoms in children and adolescents who stutter: A systematic review and meta-analysis. ***Journal of Speech, Language, and Hearing Research, 65***, 624–644. https://doi.org/10.1016/j.childyouth.2024.107924

Druker, K., Mazzucchelli, T., Hennessey, N., & Beilby, J. (2019). Parent perceptions of an integrated stuttering treatment and behavioral self-regulation program for early developmental stuttering. ***Journal of Fluency Disorders, 62***, Article 105762. https://doi.org/10.1016/j.jfludis.2019.105726

Johansson, B. (2023). ***Risk and protective factors of school bullying: A scoping review***. Örebro University.

Onslow, M. (2025). ***Stuttering and its clinical management: Twelve lectures.*** www.uts.edu.au/asrc/resources

Varlik, S. (2024). The silent shadow in primary school: The invisible face of bullying. ***Children and Youth Services Review, 166***, Article 107924.

Yaruss, J. S., Coleman, C. E., & Quesal, R. W. (2016). ***Overall Assessment of the Speaker's Experience of Stuttering (OASES-S): Ages 7–12.*** Stuttering Therapy Resources. https://stutteringtherapyresources.com/pages/oases-collections

Case study 10
Dale: choosing meaningful goals

Emma Ferris

Early intervention

Dale was born with a unilateral cleft lip and palate (CLP). He has also always had mild–moderate conductive hearing loss which he wears hearing aids for. When he was born, his family had not expected him to have any differences and did not know what a CLP was.

Theory: CLP

Theory: Hearing loss

Theory: Prevalence

Immediately after birth, Dale was diagnosed with a unilateral CLP and the cleft nurse specialist within the multidisciplinary cleft team immediately began supporting the family. As expected, Dale had two surgical operations by the plastic surgeon to repair his CLP. I am aware of how much of a burden of care lies with families whose children have CLP. There are relentless levels of appointments which start before things have even properly settled into a newborn routine for families. There is also a difficult emotional journey experienced having a baby that does not look how you expected and receive a diagnosis that changes the expectations of what being a young family is. The emotional impact is long-lasting for many families. Even though Dale is now 5, I am mindful of keeping all these factors at the forefront when making clinical decisions, giving advice to his parents and of Dale's experiences so far with medical professionals. It is common for children and their parents to have anxiety around medical appointments. I liaise closely with the psychologist who has been supporting the family recently to ensure I am up to date with his care so far and do not unnecessarily duplicate advice or assessments.

Theory: Multi-disciplinary cleft team

Theory: Surgical repair

Value: Empathy

Approach: Collaborative working

Dale's class teacher refers Dale to me. The referral includes concerns about his speech, commenting that it is difficult to understand. She also reports that his attention is very short, and his behaviour can be difficult to manage within the classroom.

DOI: 10.4324/9781003668756-13

Assessing a complex profile

Value: Holistic approach

Approach: Case history taking

I meet Dale for the first time in clinic with his mother. Assessment includes several different activities to make sure it is comprehensive, and all the information needed is gained. The first thing I do is complete a case history.

'Thank you for coming into the clinic today, it's lovely to meet you.' I look over to check that Dale is engrossed in the toys I got out for him. *'Whilst Dale plays with the toys, I would like to ask a few questions about what has happened so far for Dale. Could you tell me about his experiences of the Cleft Team so far?'*

Mum replies, *'It was all such a shock when he was born but the team have been amazing. He had his lip and palate surgery at the right times, and the surgeon is happy with how everything has healed.'* She looks relieved.

'That's really reassuring to hear.' I smile. *'I have in my notes that he has some hearing loss at the moment too?'*

'Yes, we're backwards and forwards to audiology for that every few months,' Mum says, *'It keeps fluctuating but seems to always be there. He's used to his hearing aids now and they definitely help.'*

'It's great that it's being actively managed. I appreciate it's lots of appointments though.' I look at my paper for the next question. *'How has his speech developed over time from babbling as a baby to now?'*

'He was really vocal as a baby and said his first words earlier than the children in his baby groups.' Mum has a huge smile and looks over at Dale proudly. *'He's always struggled with some sounds though ... I thought he'd grow out of it, but he hasn't.'* The smile softens and Mum becomes concerned again.

Approach: Finding balance

'Being an early talker will have been amazing for his language development,' I explain. *'It's why he's so great at telling all his stories now!'* We both look over to Dale who is playing with some action figures and narrating a whole script he has made. *'It does mean though, that he learnt to*

make sounds before his palate was repaired and so made some adaptations. His muscles weren't joined up correctly and he had a hole in the roof of his mouth. Those motor movements get engrained and stick even after the palate is repaired. His hearing difficulties would have made this harder too as he won't be able to perceive all the sounds in speech correctly.'

Clinic assessment

I explain to Mum that I need to hear Dale's speech in conversation, short phrases, single words, and then single speech sounds. I make sure the assessment is fun with lots of games and rewards for completing tasks. Dale is confident, loves the rewards, and is excited that I have a dinosaur game (his favourite animal). As I go through the activities, I keep a record of Dale's speech accuracy.

Value: Engagement

Approach: Intelligibility

Level of Assessment	Intelligibility	Specific Errors
Single Sounds	High	'sh' à [sh] ***`k' & `d' à [k] & 'd' à `k' & `d'***
Single Words	Moderate–High	Those above plus cluster errors: 'green' as 'geen' 'blue' as 'boo' 'smile' as 'mile' *'crab' as 'rab'*
Phrases	Moderate	All the above plus inconsistently: 'b' 'g' ***'v'***
Conversation	Moderate–Low	All the above plus: Mild nasal emission noted on 'p' and 'b' words.

Table 10.1 Summary of speech sound assessment for Dale

[Approach: Oro-motor examination]

I also look in Dale's mouth to note any anatomical differences. I notice that he has a pinpoint hole (fistula) in his gum into his nose as he has not yet had his alveolar bone graft. This means a very small amount of air escapes on certain sounds. Nothing else is atypical and his palate is moving well when I ask him to say 'ahhh.'

Throughout the activities, Dale's attention is good, and his language skills are typical for his age. He doesn't need many prompts to stay on task, and he engages well. When I ask Dale what he would like to play as a last game he says, '*Let's have a challenge of who can hop the most in a row.*' He enjoys being active. I talk to Mum about school's concerns around his behaviour. She does not have any concerns at home and so we agree that I will visit Dale at school.

Categorising Dale's speech errors

When assessing children, we must remember that there is a natural developmental progression with children's speech with common patterns of errors at each milestone that naturally resolve over time. If they are meeting the milestones for speech, we would not treat these errors. However, some children also sometimes have non-typical errors, which we would consider treating.

I look at my assessment findings to decide how Dale's errors fit into my knowledge of typical development as well as errors I might expect with CLP or hearing loss. His errors are consistent and can be explained as speech processes.

Error	Pattern Name	Typical Development?	Known Feature of:	
			CLP	Hearing Loss
't' as 'k' 'd' as 'g'	Backing	No	Yes	Yes
'sh'	Palatalisation	No	Yes	Yes
'green' as 'geen' 'blue' as 'boo' 'smile' as 'mile' 'crab' as 'rab'	Consonant Cluster Reduction	Yes, until age 5	No	Yes
'p' as 'b' 'k' as 'g' 'f' as 'v'	Voicing	Yes, until age 3	No	Yes
Nasal emission on 'p' and 'b'	Hypernasality	No	Yes	No

Table 10.2 Summary of Dale's speech sound error patterns

I know that Dale needs support for his speech as he is hard to understand, and this can easily lead to frustration and start to impact his language and literacy skills.

Theory: Speech sound processes

Theory: Cleft-type characteristics

School assessment

Theory: Characteristics of hearing loss

It is important to find out why Dale's behaviour and attention is so different at school compared to home and my clinic. I schedule with his class teacher to observe Dale in his classroom and whilst there I take notes:

- *Time & Lesson:* After morning break (11am). The class is finishing their time in free-choice activities and moving into a carpet-time teaching session for numeracy.
- *Free-Choice Environment:* Free-choice time is noisy. Floor is hard and furniture makes a loud noise being moved across it. The volume of children's voices is high as they speak over each other and get excited. There are 6 'stations' with different activities for them to engage with including building bricks, sand play, and colouring. A child asks Dale for his spade; he does not respond. The child then snatches the spade and Dale

shouts and throws sand in her face. The teacher comes and reminds Dale to 'share nicely.'

- *Transition:* The teacher tells the whole class they need to stop, tidy, and move to the carpet. This is delivered from the front of the class, shouting over the noise. At this point, Dale is enjoying the sand table at the back of the class. As they move to carpet time, there is lots of noise as they pack up activities and find their place on the carpet. The teacher has to go to Dale. She takes the sand toys out of his hand and walks him to the carpet. He becomes very dysregulated, tries to grab the table, shouts, and throws himself to the floor. He is partially carried to the carpet.
- *Carpet Time:* In carpet time, Dale sits at the back and fidgets. Dale does not respond to the teacher's whole-class request for them to show '4' on their fingers. The teacher speaks to Dale directly and explains what 'good listening' is. He is then asked to show '4' again. He refuses, curls up on the carpet, and picks at a loose thread.

It is concerning to see Dale struggling so much in the classroom. I consider why he may be finding it hard. The language used by the teacher was easy for him to understand, the lessons were engaging. However, the free-choice environment was very loud, and he sits at the back of the carpet for carpet time. I realise that this would make it very hard for Dale to hear with his hearing loss. He is not hearing his peers talk to him over the background noise and cannot hear the teacher clearly when she gives instructions. His first moment of hearing them is when they are outwardly frustrated with him and so he becomes confused and upset. This is not a positive pattern to continue and will impact Dale's confidence and wellbeing over time.

Prioritising and setting goals

Now I have all the information I need, goal setting is done by picking apart which errors Speech and Language Therapy (SLT) intervention can improve, and which errors are outside of my control and sit more with a surgical decision (the plastic surgeon) or hearing management decision (the audiologist). I am happy to rule out any underlying language, attention, or behaviour difficulties as the cause of his behaviour in class.

When looking at his speech sound errors, I dismiss the age-appropriate consonant cluster reduction. I also dismiss working on the hypernasality as this has the fistula as a direct cause (and can therefore only be managed surgically).

Palatalisation makes less impact on his intelligibility, and I know that working on his articulation for this will be easier and more effective when he is a little older. Voicing could be due to a delay in typical development but is more likely to be due to his hearing loss. This could be a goal, but it is inconsistent and only heard at phrase level and conversation.

However, backing is not typical and could be due to either of his difficulties. This does affect his intelligibility and is more significant given his name is Dale (produced by him as 'Gale') which he explains makes him embarrassed. Quality of life, access to education, and wellbeing are all at the forefront when prioritising children between each other but also selecting which elements to work on first. Being able to say his name correctly is therefore a key outcome for Dale.

[Value: Person-centred]

His hearing environment is also a significant barrier to his social communication, play, and learning, and could easily become a source of social, emotional, and mental health concern. This aspect of intervention will not be working with Dale directly. Instead, I plan to work with his teachers and provide training. Simple strategies such as moving him toward the front of the carpet, gaining his attention before speaking, trying to minimise background noise, and using visuals to support spoken language will reduce many of the barriers he has to accessing the communication environment and have a significant impact.

[Approach: Inclusive environment]

I identify two strands to my intervention:

1. Increasing speech sound accuracy and intelligibility.
    a. For Dale to be able to use /t/ and /d/ in his speech.
2. Improving his access to the learning environment.
    a. For staff to modify their communication to ensure Dale's inclusion.

Reflections

I enjoy working with complex children. There is a duty as the SLT to be informed and up to date with the evidence base and literature relating to their speech, language, and communication needs. The detective work needed to complete a thorough investigation (assessment) and then accurately analyse that data is more challenging. Children with CLP have additional risk factors and a complex profile to consider due to medical diagnoses and the involvement of a multi-disciplinary team (MDT) measuring overall outcomes through a medical model of care. School-age children also sit within an educational MDT and are measured against educational attainment.

The decisions I make as Dale's SLT need to integrate both the medical and educational, ensuring outcomes for both are supported. It is important that I do not over-medicalise Dale and remember that he is a complex young child who needs to be considered holistically. Goals need to be set to break down barriers to his current daily life and wellbeing.

Dale will likely need more support in the future from an SLT as he makes progress against these goals and develops as a person. The process will continue, as his speech, language, and communication skills evolve.

Questions for reflection and discussion

1. What might it be like for a family when their baby is born with unexpected medical complications?
2. What might it feel like to have hearing loss? How might it impact your interactions with others?
3. Why is information sharing important between families, MDT members (medical and/or educational), and the SLT?
4. How can SLTs support teachers to improve the communication environment within the classroom?
5. What gives children a good quality of life?
6. What are the impacts for children of having a speech, language, or communication difficulty?

Further reading

Bowen, C. (2023). ***Children's speech sound disorders*** (3rd ed.). Wiley Blackwell.

CLAPA (Cleft Lip and Palate Association): www.clapa.com

CLEFT (International Development Organization): www.cleft.org.uk

Speech and Language UK: www.speechandlanguage.org.uk

NDCS (National Deaf Children's Society): www.ndcs.org.uk

ICF (International Classification of Function, Disability and Health): www.who.int/standards/classifications/international-classification-of-functioning-disability-and-health

Further information

Theories

Characteristics of hearing loss: children with conductive hearing loss are unable to perceive certain sound frequencies (dependent on their hearing levels). Speech sounds are all at slightly different frequencies, meaning some are heard clearly, and others not. Children learn words and which sounds are in them through their environment. As they mis-hear, so they mis-store those words, causing them to say them incorrectly in their own speech.

CLP: cleft lip and/or palate occurs during weeks 3–9 of embryological development, where the face and palate structures come together and fuse ('zip up') down the midline. An incomplete fusing process causes a cleft, which is a gap/lack of boundary between the oral and nasal cavity. This gap also means that muscles that would usually be attached at the midline are not. The cleft could be solely at the lip (cleft lip), solely at the palate (cleft palate), or go through from lip to palate (cleft lip and palate). CLP affects airflow for speech as well as eating, drinking, and swallowing (NHS, 2023).

Cleft-type characteristics: cleft-type characteristics in speech are due to a structural difficulty which the child has no control over. They can be caused by the child actively trying to compensate for the structural anomaly as they learn to say those sounds before cleft repair. Some difficulties, such as resonance, children cannot compensate for and so passively appear in their speech. Around 50% of children with CLP need SLT intervention at some point in their journey and the average age when a child with CLP becomes intelligible to others is nearly 8 years old compared to the average of 3 years old in a non-CLP population. Children aged 3 with CLP are typically not understood by strangers (Seifert et al., 2021).

Hearing loss: conductive hearing loss is a form of hearing impairment that occurs when sounds cannot pass effectively from the outer to inner ear due to a blockage in the middle ear. In children with CLP this is due to recurrent ear infections in the middle ear. Children with CLP are more at risk of this as the muscles in the soft palate (affected by the cleft) are also responsible for helping the eustachian tube (the tube linking your middle ear to the back of your throat) to regulate the pressure and support drainage of any fluid/infection from the middle ear (NDCS, n.d.).

Multi-disciplinary cleft team has a core number of professionals included: plastic surgeon, maxilla-facial surgeon, clinical psychologist, cleft nurse specialist, audiologist and Speech and Language Therapist. Centre outcomes are monitored and compared nationally in the UK via CRANE (Cleft Registry and Audit NEtwork).

Prevalence: around 1 in 700 babies born in the UK are born with a CLP and so it is a relatively common occurrence. Of those children, 22% have a unilateral cleft lip and palate like Dale (CRANE, 2021). Sometimes a cleft lip can be identified on the 20-week anomaly screening scan during pregnancy. Whilst some types of CLP have a genetic component, many do not.

Speech sound processes: there is a typical developmental pattern to speech sound acquisition and accuracy, meaning that the expected error patterns gradually reduce as the child develops. If children resolve them at the expected milestones they are classed as age appropriate. If they miss the milestones, they are considered delayed. Some children have patterns that are not seen in typical development, and this is considered non-typical. All error patterns have a name to describe the process happening:

- Voicing: the vocal cords innervate and vibrate during production of the sound, making it voiced, but should remain still (voiceless).
- Backing: sounds produced at the back of the mouth with the back of the tongue are produced at the front with the front of the tongue.
- Consonant cluster reduction: words with multiple consonants together as a blend are produced with less consonants.
- Palatalisation: the sound is produced by using the sides of the tongue against the teeth to modify the airflow, rather than the front middle of the tongue against the gum.

Surgical repair: there are standard timings for CLP surgery. These are conformed to unless there is a medical reason not to. Lip and hard palate repair occur at 4 months, soft palate repair at 10 months. When dental development reaches a certain point (just before permanent canines erupt), children then have an alveolar bone graft operation to repair the final element of the CLP – a fistula (hole) from the gum into the nasal cavity that is not repaired in the earlier surgeries (NHS, 2023).

Approaches

Case history taking: this involves interviewing the primary caregiver to gain greater understanding of how the child has developed to date. This includes developmental milestones in motor, sensory, communication, eating/drinking, and play skills. For children with a medical history, it would also consider diagnoses and their management.

Collaborative working: due to the complex nature of CLP, children and their families receive support from a wide MDT. For this to be effective, members of the team must communicate their professional opinions, knowledge, and action plans to avoid repetition of advice or assessments and overwhelm of extra appointments for the family. This ensures effective and efficient treatment.

Finding balance: the diagnostic process for SLT cannot focus only on the negatives and deficits a patient has. A rounded view of their communication profile is required, and so strengths must also be highlighted. This improves clinical decision making but also avoids sounding overly negative.

Inclusive environment: the SLT will often consider the child's surroundings and advise others, such as teachers, on how to make the setting as accessible as possible.

Intelligibility: this is a measurable outcome for communication. Instead of focussing on specific sound or word accuracy, it considers how easy the speaker is to understand overall. This is seen as a more functional social-model measure of communication.

Oro-motor examination: this aids the therapist in understanding the person's physiology and which speech sounds and qualities they are capable and not capable of producing. In CLP, the oro-motor exam should consider mobility and accuracy of movement of the lips, soft palate, and tongue. It should also consider anatomical differences that could impact those movements and airflow such as teeth alignment, jaw alignment, and any fistulae.

Values

Empathy: the breadth of the MDT and multiple early interventions mean that families have regular medical appointments in addition to the typical demands of having a young baby/child. These appointments are sometimes called 'burden of care.' It is important to empathise with the impact this has on parents' wellbeing and ability to engage.

Engagement: children respond best when they are happy and interested. Games and rewards are integrated into clinical appointments to reduce the child's anxiety and increase their attention. When activities integrate their interests, this is further enhanced and supports rapport building. A more fun, relaxed environment also provides more natural communication samples and opportunities.

Holistic approach: children must be supported as a whole person, considering their wellbeing and social factors, not just medical factors. This enables professionals to make meaningful difference to the quality of their lives with.

Person-centred: value must be given to each child's wishes and desires for treatment. Goals should be selected in collaboration with the child and family to ensure it addresses their needs. This may mean that therapists deviate from the textbook goal selection process.

References

CRANE (Cleft Registry and Audit Network). (2021). ***CRANE database 2021 annual report***. Retrieved 29 June 2025, from www.crane-database.org.uk/reports/crane-database-2021-annual-report/

NDCS (National Deaf Children's Society). (n.d.). ***NDCS***. Retrieved 29 August 2025, from www.ndcs.org.uk

NHS (National Health Service). (2023). ***Cleft lip and palate: Treatment***. Retrieved 29 June 2025, from www.nhs.uk/conditions/cleft-lip-and-palate/treatment/

Seifert, M., Davies, A., Harding, S., McLeod, S., & Wren, Y. (2021). Intelligibility in 3-year-olds with cleft lip and/or palate using the intelligibility in context scale: Findings from the Cleft Collective Cohort Study. ***The Cleft Palate-Craniofacial Journal, 58***(9), 1178–1189. https://doi.org/10.1177/1055665620986567

Part 3

Interdisciplinary working in Speech and Language Therapy

Case study 11
Samuel: 'they can't possibly cope at home'

Elissa Manzi

Meeting Samuel

I meet Samuel whilst working as a specialist speech and language therapist on a stroke rehabilitation ward. He has recently been transferred from the local acute hospital, where he was admitted after a left Middle Cerebral Artery (MCA) infarct. I was asked to assess him due to communication difficulties caused by aphasia.

Theory: Left Middle Cerebral Artery Infarct

Theory: Aphasia

Samuel's past medical history includes depression and diabetes, which are risk factors for strokes. He has also experienced declining vision prior to his stroke because of cataracts. His visual difficulties have been further exacerbated by the stroke, resulting in significant right visual field loss. Samuel is fully mobile but finds it difficult to safely navigate around the ward due to his vision and often bumps into things.

During our first meeting, I spend time getting to know Samuel before carrying out an assessment of his language abilities.

Approach: Initial assessment

I walk into his bay on the ward, whiteboard in hand. Samuel is sitting in his chair. He looks up.

Approach: Supported communication

'*Hi there*', I say, waving gently and point to my name badge. '*I'm Elissa. I'm a speech and language therapist*'. As I say this, I write: '*Elissa – speech*' in big letters on the whiteboard and show it to him.

Samuel responds, '*Ah! Speaky... uh, speak, you right!*'

I nod, smiling, and sit down beside him. I explain, '*I'm here to help with talking... and understanding. We'll work together. Is that okay?*' '*Yes, yes*', Samuel says excitedly, '*Very wobbly, the words, they- zip! Gone and then gone but I'm good*'.

DOI: 10.4324/9781003668756-15

'That's okay', I say smiling, *'We'll figure it out together. I'd love to get to know you a bit more. What do you enjoy? Any hobbies?'*

Samuel gestures to his iPod and says, *'Yes yes, here we go and the big sound'*.

'Music! Me too!' I say as I writing *'Music♫'* on the whiteboard, *'What sort of music do you like?'* I write the options *'pop, rock, jazz, blues, country, classical'* on the whiteboard in large letters.

Samuel looks at the options carefully and points to classical, pop and rock. He then shows me that he has been listening to Queen and Pink Floyd on his iPod.

'Nice!' I say enthusiastically, *'I like Bruce Springsteen... Billy Joel... Mumford and Sons.'* I write the names out slowly on the board as I say them and point to each word. *'Do you like those?'*

Samuel wrinkles his nose dramatically, *'Nooo, no, no boring is for me'*, he says, *'No jump!'* He mimes falling asleep, snoring.

I laugh with him, pretending to be shocked, *'Hey! That's rude!'* I say, *'Bruce is the Boss!'*

Samuel grins and shrugs in response to this.

'Fair enough!' I say, gesturing *'you win.'* I continue, *'So, how are you feeling? About being here, the stroke?'* I write down key words.

Samuel's expression softens. He pauses, searching for words, *'Strange brain not me. All fuzzy.'*

I soften my expression as well, saying, *'Thank you for sharing that. That's really important.*

I want to help. I'm here to support your communication. We'll work on talking, listening, reading, and writing – together'. I show him a picture board with simple icons representing ear, mouth, pen, book. I point to each.

Due to Samuel's very limited vision, it is difficult for him to see me, or the resources I have brought with me to support his aphasia. This means it is harder for him to express himself as he finds it challenging to use pictures and writing; things that often support communication for people with aphasia. It helps when I write and draw in large print on the whiteboard. Establishing Samuel's interests and feelings in our initial meeting allowed me to build rapport, before launching in to more formal assessment.

Value: Building rapport

Based on my initial interaction and subsequent assessments, Samuel has moderate Wernicke's aphasia. He has difficulties understanding what others are saying, particularly when they give him lots of information or when information is lengthy or complex. His speech is fluent but the words he does use are not always the words he is intending to use. This means his speech does not always make sense to the listener. A further complication is that he is not always aware of his communication difficulties. This leads to Samuel understandably experiencing frustration at not being understood by other staff on the hospital ward. He tells me that he feels restricted and misunderstood by others in the hospital ward environment.

Theory: Wernicke's aphasia

Working with Samuel

As I continue to work with Samuel in the subsequent days, he is able to recognise my voice and seems to feel comfortable during our speech and language therapy sessions. Within the sessions, he often relies heavily on auditory and tactile cues, due to visual loss. We focus our therapy on finding ways to successfully communicate and establish total communication strategies which benefit his understanding and expression. I also spend time advising his best friend on how best to communicate with him.

Theory: Total communication

Approach: Training others

I talk to Samuel about what he would like to achieve from our therapy. His main priority is to return to his flat, where he has lived alone for many years. He dislikes being in a hospital environment and wants to return to the comfort of his home, with access to treasured belongings such as his vinyl collection.

Approach: Person-centred therapy

Approach: Adapting communication

The multi-disciplinary team (MDT) shares concerns regarding Samuel's communication and cognition, particularly his ability to access help at home in emergency situations, and complete daily tasks such as personal care and shopping. It is crucial that Samuel is not excluded from discharge decisions, and I identify the communication strategies that will support him to be involved in decision-making and to express his opinions. Helpful strategies for Samuel include giving him time to express himself, modifying the communication environment (e.g. reducing background noise), simplifying and rephrasing information and encouraging all types of communication, e.g. gesture and other non-verbal communication.

Theory: Mental capacity assessments

Samuel is involved through the whole discharge planning process and the communication strategies outlined next are used to support him throughout. A mental capacity assessment is carried out due to concerns from the MDT to determine his ability to decide where he will live when leaving hospital. It is important to ensure he is supported in his communication throughout this assessment and my role as a speech and language therapist is crucial here.

The following practicable steps are taken to ensure Samuel is supported during this assessment.

MDT preparation and support

Value: Interprofessional communication

I work alongside social worker, Rachel, to facilitate the assessment. This ensures there is appropriate communication support alongside all the relevant discharge information. I meet with Rachel beforehand to plan our assessment.

Rachel begins, *'We need to schedule Samuel's capacity assessment. What's our starting point?'*

'Let's block out an hour to avoid rushing', I suggest, *'We don't need to use the whole time and we should be aware of Samuel's fatigue. I'll bring visual aids like picture cards and a yes/no board. Can we see if we can book the day room so that we have a quiet space?'*

'Perfect. I'll prepare discharge-related info and clear up any questions we need answered,' says Rachel, *'How should we work together during the assessment? Shall we split it half and half?'*

'My main role will be to support his communication,' I say, *'This means ensuring he understands the information presented and can express himself. You have more knowledge and expertise about the discharge itself and so can answer any queries about that.'*

'Got it,' Rachel says, before adding, *'And if he needs a break or uses visuals, I'll pause and clarify practical implications.'*

'Exactly,' I agree, *'Also, I've prepped short guidance for the rest of the MDT – how to slow down language, use simple sentences, cue pauses. I can send you a copy if helpful.'*

Rachel responds enthusiastically, *'Yes please! Great. After the assessment, I'll draft the outcome section with his expressed wishes and hand it over for you to note communication methods used.'*

I add, *'Yes, and if we need a follow-up slot to revisit anything, we can build that in. We may not be able to get through everything in one session. Does that cover everything for now?'*

Assessing Samuel's mental capacity

I meet Samuel in a private, quiet room on the ward, away from the shared bay where he's been staying. It's important to reduce distractions as much as possible, especially given the complexity of the decision ahead. The room is calm, without background noise. I want him to feel comfortable, and to be able to focus and express himself fully.

Approach: Adapting the communication environment

Before starting the mental capacity assessment, I take time to re-establish how best to support Samuel's communication. In previous sessions, I have learned that he responds well to large images, bold single-word text and simple language. Today, I have brought a pack of picture cards and photos, each showing key elements of daily living: front door, cooker, stairs, phone and large written words beneath.

I sit across from Samuel so he can see me clearly. Keeping my tone warm and steady, I say, *'Samuel, we're going to talk about whether going home is the right option for you now.'* I pause to watch his response.

Samuel nods quickly, and gestures toward himself with his thumb, saying, *'We see home, yes. In the moment home, yes.'*

His speech is fluent but often contains jargon or irrelevant words, typical of Wernicke's aphasia. I stay focused on the intent behind his words. I hold up a photo of his front door that we took during a visit to his property last week.

'This is your front door. Do you remember our visit?' I ask.

He grins, *'My blue door and I talk with a lot of others about the door, to go home.'*

'Yes,' I smile, *'We walked around your flat. I'm going to show you some pictures from that day, and we can talk about what felt easy, or what felt hard.'*

We look through photos together: the stairs to get to the flat, the bathroom, the cooker in this kitchen. For each, I present one image at a time, using short, clear phrases, and giving plenty of time for him to respond. I watch his gestures, his facial expressions, and encourage him to point or use the word cards as needed.

When we come to the stairs, I ask: *'Do you feel safe going up and down these stairs?'*

Samuel frowns slightly, *'Yes yes, bit... hmm... slow and not working always over here on the day.'* He points to his eyes and gestures to vision on his right side.

I note his hesitation. *'It can be difficult to see on the right side?'* I ask.

'*Yes, yes, slow down,*' he says, placing emphasis on the word '*slow.*'

Throughout, I repeat key questions as needed, paraphrasing to aid comprehension. If Samuel seems unsure, I offer simplified alternatives or point to visuals. I never rush. We take breaks. Samuel asks for a drink halfway through, and we pause for ten minutes.

Samuel's close friend, David, sits beside him quietly. With Samuel's prior permission, I have invited him to attend. Occasionally, David checks in gently, asking, '*You okay, Sam?*'

Samuel touches his hand briefly, '*Yeah... good good.*'

David's presence clearly comforts him.

I ask, '*Samuel, what would happen if you went home and something went wrong?*' This is an important question and something we have spoken about before, with the occupational therapist on the ward.

Samuel looks down, then gestures a fall with his hand and says, '*Bang hurt. Phone them and then talking away but no,*' he gestures to mouth, '*and then we talk and nobody, nobody comes.*'

I nod slowly, '*Yes. That's a risk. You might need help but not be able to talk on the phone. But you understand that. What will help?*'

He points to a picture of a pendant alarm in front of him, '*people come.*' He points to David.

We discuss options for assisted living and home care. In this moment, with support, visual prompts, enough time and emotional reassurance, Samuel clearly expresses his wish, shows understanding of the risks and is able to weigh them against his preferences.

The outcome

In Samuel's case, a comprehensive assessment demonstrates his capacity to make informed decisions about his discharge, and he decides to be discharged home. He acknowledges potential risks and is agreeable to external support being provided in order to mitigate these risks.

Despite the outcome of the mental capacity assessment, some MDT members continue to express concerns about Samuel's discharge, questioning the validity of the capacity assessment due to his aphasia.

In a mid-morning MDT meeting, the team are discussing discharge planning for Samuel, and I update the team about the outcome of the recent mental capacity assessment, and Samuel's decision to go home with support. One of the nurse's frowns slightly and says, *'I just don't see how he could possibly cope at home. He can barely get his words out. How's he going to call for help, or tell someone what he needs?'*

One of the rehabilitation assistants agrees, *'Exactly. I know he said he wanted to go home, but is he really understanding what that means? It doesn't feel right to send him home when he can't even hold a proper conversation.'*

Rachel the social worker gently interjects, *'He was assessed and found to have capacity. It's about whether he can understand, retain, weigh up and communicate his decision – not whether we agree with the choice.'*

I add, calmly and with a reassuring tone, *'I hear your concerns. It's understandable. We all want Samuel to be safe. But throughout the capacity assessment, I supported his communication. We used visual aids, a yes/no board, and gave him plenty of processing time. And he was able to clearly express his reasons for wanting to go home.'* I pause, making eye contact around the room, *'He understood the risks and could explain how he'd manage. It wasn't a quick or easy conversation – but it was a valid one.'*

The nurse is still doubtful, *'But what if something happens and he can't tell anyone? Wouldn't that come back to us?'*

'We've thought about that too,' I say, *'The discharge plan includes daily care visits, and a charity is supporting him with communication tools at home. He will have a pendant alarm linked to his neighbour. So, we're not sending him home without support. We've done what we can to support Samuel to make his own decision and put things in place to reduce any risk.'*

Rachel adds, *'And remember, having aphasia doesn't mean someone lacks capacity. It just means we need to adapt how we communicate. Which we did.'*

The healthcare assistant considers this for a moment and says, *'I guess... I just worry. He's lovely. I'd hate for him to feel isolated.'*

I nod, *'And that's completely valid. We all care. Let's keep working together to make sure the support around him is as strong as it can be. There are local aphasia support groups we will tell him about too. But ultimately, he has the right to make this choice.'*

Reflections

A multi-disciplinary approach

Multi-disciplinary team (MDT) working is essential in stroke care to provide comprehensive, person-centred rehabilitation that addresses the complex physical, cognitive, emotional and social needs of each individual. Collaborative input from a range of professionals can ensure timely, coordinated care and improve outcomes across all stages of recovery. For individuals with aphasia, MDT working is crucial to ensure communication needs are recognised and supported by all team members throughout the care pathway. Speech and language therapists play a key role in enabling individuals to participate meaningfully in their care, while collaboration with other professionals ensures adaptations are made to support the individual across all disciplines, thereby maximising independence and respecting patient autonomy.

Effective discharge planning necessitates collaboration between healthcare professionals. In Samuel's case, key MDT members involved were nurses, social workers, occupational therapists and speech and language therapists.

Challenging misconceptions about aphasia

Despite the outcome of the mental capacity assessment in this case, some MDT members continue to express concerns about Samuel's discharge, questioning the validity of the capacity assessment due to his aphasia. One member of staff states he *'couldn't possibly'* go home due to his level of aphasia.

Such reactions are unfortunately not uncommon and, in my experience, people with aphasia report how they are often dismissed and misunderstood, or that assumptions are made about them and their abilities by others. This underscores the presence of unconscious biases, where communication impairments are mistakenly equated with cognitive deficits and a lack of ability.

Addressing unconscious biases toward individuals with aphasia is crucial for fostering an inclusive and empathetic society. Aphasia impairs language abilities without affecting intelligence. However, many people mistakenly equate speech and language disorders with cognitive deficits, leading to social exclusion and reduced opportunities for those affected. By recognising and challenging these biases, we can promote better communication practices, ensure equitable access to services and support the autonomy and dignity of individuals with aphasia. There is a lack of public awareness of aphasia but also a need for more education and training within healthcare, so that all healthcare professionals feel confident and comfortable supporting the needs of people with aphasia or know where to access guidance and support.

Organisations such as the UK-based Tavistock Trust for Aphasia, Aphasia Support Network and Aphasia Re-Connect demonstrate the positive impact of inclusive approaches, such as creating accessible environments and involving people with aphasia in decision-making processes.

In this case, Samuel's capacity was not assumed by ward staff; quite the opposite. It is essential that relevant training on the principles of mental capacity, as well as education about aphasia, are provided across the MDT. The need for practicable steps to be taken is also emphasised, considering how this may look for someone with aphasia. This case also emphasises the importance of speech and language therapy involvement in mental capacity assessments for people with communication difficulties. It is important to note that every person and every presentation is individual; two people may have experienced a left MCA stroke and both present with aphasia and yet the practicable steps needed to support them may be very different. It is important to take the time to get to know the individual involved, and how best they communicate.

Ensuring support is in place

It is known from sociological studies that living at home alone increases risk of loneliness and adverse physical and mental health outcomes (Snell, 2017). Remaining socially connected is essential to support wellbeing (Hersh et al., 2024). Therefore, it was important to ensure Samuel was well connected in the community, should he want this. On discussion, Samuel was keen to be directed to any community support and opportunities to socialise. He was directed to the local peer-led aphasia café, and we offered to organise his first visit with a member of the community stroke team.

I worked closely with the occupational therapist and social worker and it was arranged that Samuel would receive twice daily care visits, delivery of shopping through the Red Cross, support with cleaning his property and referral to third sector support such as the Stroke Association and a local charity for the visually impaired. He was also provided with a pendant alarm, and use of the alarm was trialled on the ward, where it was established that Samuel could use this appropriately and safely.

Central to Samuel's case is the emphasis on person-centred care, respecting his preferences and involving him actively in the decision-making process. Advocacy played a pivotal role, ensuring that his voice was heard and his rights protected. Speech and language therapists are instrumental in facilitating communication and advocating for the needs of individuals with aphasia.

Questions for reflection and discussion

1. What communication strategies might be beneficial to support somebody with fluent aphasia?
2. What is the role of the speech and language therapist in supporting mental capacity assessments?
3. Consider how people with aphasia may experience conversations about discharge planning and mental capacity assessments?
4. How can speech and language therapists ensure members of the MDT feel confident in supporting the communication of people with aphasia, across all stages of the care pathway?
5. How can we make the discharge process more accessible for people with aphasia?
6. What support could be accessed from community or third sector services, to support with safe and person-centred discharge planning?

Further reading

Aphasia Reconnect: https://aphasiareconnect.org/

Aphasia Support Network: www.aphasiasupport.org/

Borrett, S., & Gould, L. J. (2020). Mental capacity assessment with people with aphasia: understanding the role of the speech and language therapist. ***Aphasiology***, ***35***(11), 1463–1481.

Hinckley, J., & Jayes, M. (2023). Person-centred care for people with aphasia: tools for shared decision-making. ***Frontiers in Rehabilitation Sciences***, ***4***, 1236534. https://doi.org/10.3389/fresc.2023.1236534

Tavistock Trust for Aphasia: https://aphasiatavistocktrust.org/

Further information

Theories

Aphasia is a language processing disorder. It does not affect intellect but can affect any or all language modalities, i.e. comprehension, expression (such as finding words and putting sentences together), reading and writing.

Left Middle Cerebral Artery infarct is a type of stroke impacting the largest cerebral artery, preventing blood and oxygen flow to parts of the left hemisphere of the brain, including areas responsible for language comprehension and expression.

Mental capacity assessments help to determine a person's understanding of their condition and their ability to make a particular decision at a particular time. They are carried out if there is doubt that the person is able to make the decision, due to an illness or impairment (NHS, 2025).

Total communication uses all means of communication and places equal value on each modality of language, e.g. gesture, writing, drawing and facial expression, which can often increase the success of communication exchanges for people with aphasia.

Wernicke's aphasia (sometimes known as fluent or receptive aphasia) can result in fluent speech that includes jargon or neologisms (i.e. words that are not recognisable as real words). Individuals with this aphasia type often produce syntactically correct language but can lack insight into their errors (Hallowell, 2017).

Approaches

Adapting communication for people with aphasia involves adjusting how we share and receive information so they can fully participate in conversations. This might include speaking slowly and clearly, using simple sentences, supporting speech with visuals or gestures, and giving extra time for responses.

Adapting the communication environment: practical considerations such as reducing background noise, removing distractions, considering positioning and lighting can aid individuals with aphasia in understanding what is said to them and expressing themselves.

Initial assessment includes time for getting to know the individual, building rapport and taking a case history, as well as the use of specific assessment tools focused on aspects of communication.

Person-centred therapy is based around the individual's priorities, needs and values, to ensure that therapy goals are relevant and meaningful to them.

Supported communication includes providing information for people with aphasia in an accessible format, accompanying speech, with other methods such as written words, images and gesture (Pound et al., 2000).

Training others to communicate with individuals with aphasia is an important aspect of therapy and can increase the success of interactions, reducing frustration for the person with aphasia and their family, friends and carers.

Values

Building rapport involves recognising the person, not the disability; it means focusing on their individuality, strengths and experiences rather than just their communication difficulties. This can help people with aphasia feel more comfortable and confident in interactions.

Interprofessional communication is important in providing coordinated and effective care. It relies on clarity, respect and collaboration to ensure that everyone involved works toward shared goals in the best interest of the individual.

References

Hallowell, B. (2017). ***Aphasia and other acquired neurogenic language disorders: A guide for clinical excellence*** (1st ed.). Plural Publishing.

Hersh, D., Williamson, C., Brogan, E., & Stanley, M. (2024). It's day to day problems: Experiences of people with aphasia who live alone. ***International Journal of Speech-Language Pathology, 26***(3), 367–379. https://doi.org/10.1080/17549507.2023.2208317

NHS (National Health Service). (2025, June 6). ***Mental Capacity Act***. Retrieved June 6, 2025 ,from www.nhs.uk/conditions/mental-capacity-act/

Pound, C., Parr, S., Lindsay, J., & Woolf, C. (2000). ***Beyond aphasia***. Routledge.

Snell, K. D. M. (2017). The rise of living alone and loneliness in history. ***Social History, 42***(1), 2–28. https://doi.org/10.1080/03071022.2016.1256089

Case study 12
Diego: dealing with obstacles as a stutterer

Veronica Fierro

Reason for referral

I am a bilingual (English/Spanish) speech-language therapist (SLT) working in a public elementary school when I am informed that a parent (mother) is seeking services for her child (Diego) due to stuttering. This is Diego's first year at this school. Although referrals occasionally come directly from parents, it is more common to receive them from teachers who have concerns about their students. I am surprised that I have not heard from Diego's teacher first, especially when it pertains to a student who stutters. I called Diego's mother to obtain more information and to ask her to come to the school to sign paperwork to give me permission to evaluate Diego (if warranted). When I meet Diego's mother, she expresses concerns about the reemergence of his stuttering. She notes that Diego had exhibited disfluent speech in early childhood, but it had *'mostly gone away'* by age four. He has never received speech-language therapy, and in his previous school, minor disfluencies were noted, but these were attributed to his bilingualism and that he was still learning how to speak in English. Recently, however, stuttering behaviors have intensified, especially during emotionally charged conversations, in new social situations, and when switching between languages.

Theory: Stuttering

Approach: Case history

Approach: Consent to evaluate

Theory: Second language acquisition

During the intake interview Diego's mother says: *'He (Diego) used to talk nonstop as a little boy, always in Spanish. But now, sometimes, he just... shuts down mid-sentence or looks like he's fighting with his own words.'*

Background information

Diego's mother reports that she and her husband are biologically Diego's aunt and uncle, and that they adopted him when he was three years old. Diego lost his biological

DOI: 10.4324/9781003668756-16

mother to suicide when he was just two years old and a few months after her death, his biological father was incarcerated due to criminal charges of drug possession and trafficking. As a result, Diego was placed in foster care. Diego's biological father was encouraged to put Diego up for adoption, and after Diego's biological father made the decision to terminate his parental rights, Diego's now adoptive mother and father made the request to adopt him and become his legal guardians. Diego is aware that he is adopted, that his mother died (although he was not told how she died), and that his father is in prison. He also has a biological sister who was adopted by Diego's grandparents, although they chose not to adopt him. Diego's adoptive mother told me that Diego experienced significant trauma prior to his adoption, including neglect and inconsistent caregiving in early childhood. She feels that while his adoptive family has been supportive and nurturing of Diego, the early trauma has had lasting emotional effects. Diego's adoptive mother reports that he experiences fluency breakdowns triggered by anxiety, emotional stress, and when he switches between English (school language) and Spanish (home language). He avoids speaking in class and with unfamiliar adults.

Diego's mother says: *'He gets really upset if people look at him funny when he's trying to say something. He'd rather stay quiet than feel judged.'*

'I don't understand what's causing him to stutter so much. Is it because of what he's gone through? Or is it because we speak mostly Spanish at home, and he's expected to speak only in English at school?' She adds.

Despite these challenges, Diego demonstrates strong academic capabilities, especially in written expression. According to his classroom teacher, Mrs. Evans, Diego is introspective and thoughtful but socially withdrawn. Mrs. Evans notes that Diego rarely participates verbally in class, despite being one of the top-performing students. When he does speak, his utterances are typically short, which is why she has not taken notice of his stuttering. She states that he avoids group activities and spends recess alone.

The thorough case history I obtain from Diego's mother reveals the multiple adverse childhood experiences Diego has experienced due to early childhood trauma and disrupted attachment. The behaviors that Diego exhibits in school indicate a pattern of internalized anxiety and low self-esteem, exacerbated by his stuttering and traumatic history. The increase in his disfluent speech, combined with his early trauma history, indicate that his stuttering is not due to second language acquisition but is likely multifactorial.

Theory: Adverse childhood experiences

Theory: Multifactorial causes of stuttering

Assessment procedures and results

When I first meet Diego, he appears shy and withdrawn. He frequently avoids eye contact and hesitates before speaking, especially when unfamiliar topics are introduced. He tells me he has feelings of frustration and embarrassment when speaking, particularly in the classroom.

'*I try to talk, but my words get stuck... like they're hiding from me.*' Diego says.

I assess Diego's speech and language abilities in English and Spanish. To determine his frequency and type of disfluencies, I assess him using the Stuttering Severity Instrument (SSI-4). Other assessment tools that I utilize for the assessment include an oral mechanism exam, a language sample analysis using conversational and reading tasks, an informal receptive and expressive language screener, and observations of Diego in the classroom and during recess. Table 12.1 demonstrates the key findings of Diego's assessment. Diego exhibits stuttering in both languages, with slightly more disfluencies in English—his school language. He does not demonstrate any oral-facial abnormalities, and his receptive and expressive language abilities are within the normal range. Diego's academic and cognitive abilities are in the upper normal range, based on the evaluation by the school psychologist. Findings by the school's social worker regarding Diego's social-emotional abilities reveal feelings of frustration and embarrassment, as well as anxiety and depressive symptoms.

Approach: Stuttering Severity Instrument (SSI-4)

Approach: Comprehensive speech-language assessment

Frequency and Type of Disfluencies	Moderate to severe stuttering with part- and whole-word repetitions, prolongations, and blocks. Secondary behaviors (eye blinking, head nodding, lip tension) are also observed. Disfluencies noted in both languages, but slightly more pronounced in English.
Situational Variability	Increased disfluencies noted in high-pressure environments such as reading aloud in class or speaking to unfamiliar individuals.
Communication Attitudes	Diego expresses frustration and embarrassment related to his speech. He reports feeling anxious when speaking and notes that his peers mock his stutter.
Emotional and Behavioral Indicators	Observations and checklists indicate signs of anxiety, avoidance behaviors, and depressive symptoms.

Table 12.1 Key findings of Diego's assessment

Intervention plan

Approach: Multi-disciplinary

Approach: Trauma-informed care

Given the complex interplay between trauma and stuttering in this case, a multi-disciplinary and a trauma-informed approach are adopted. According to Yairi and Seery (2023), the therapeutic objectives for a school-aged child should focus on increasing fluency, reducing stuttering, and improving emotional and social adjustment. So the goals for speech-language therapy that I develop for Diego in consultation with his parents include: 1) to reduce the frequency and severity of stuttering; 2) to increase Diego's confidence in verbal expression; and 3) to develop strategies for self-advocacy and communication resilience.

Value: Acceptance

Approach: Stuttering therapy strategies

I explain and reinforce to Diego that it is okay to stutter. During therapy sessions, we practice strategies for fluent speech, strategies to manage his stuttering during the times he cannot produce fluent speech, and voluntary stuttering in role-play situations. Since I am also bilingual in Spanish and English, one of my objectives is also to validate Diego's bilingual identity. Therefore, therapy includes both English and Spanish contexts. We practice scenarios in both English and Spanish, and I encourage him to code-switch when it is helpful for him, not only for linguistic factors (e.g., word retrieval) but also to ease his stuttering. After a few weeks of therapy, Diego reports improvements in his communication abilities.

Diego begins: *'It feels better when I know I can take my time. I'm not in a race with my words.'*

'I used to think I was broken... now I know I just talk different sometimes, and that's okay,' he explains during the mid-therapy session.

Emotional vocabulary and regulation strategies are integrated into sessions. I tell Diego, *'We don't just work on speech. We work on feeling safe with speech.'* Psychosocial support is also provided to Diego by the school's counselor, which includes weekly therapy sessions focused on processing trauma, building self-esteem, and developing coping strategies, as well as the use of adapted cognitive behavioral therapy (CBT) techniques that are applicable to children. Furthermore, I introduce Diego to a small, peer group facilitated by me that includes other children in the school who stutter to promote social interaction, reduce isolation, and practice the strategies they are learning during individual interventions sessions.

Approach: Cognitive Behavioral Therapy (CBT)

Approach: Group therapy

I also include Diego's parents and teachers in his intervention plan. I provide them all with information on stuttering and I explain to them that, at his age, Diego's stuttering is not going to go away, and that it is more important to focus on increasing his communication abilities instead of focusing on him obtaining fluent speech. I collaborate with Mrs. Evans on the implementation of classroom accommodations, and I encourage Diego's parents to continue to maintain their use of Spanish at home. In addition, I provide Diego's parents with parent coaching sessions in which I educate them on the use of supportive communication strategies and how to reduce the demands placed on Diego to communicate.

Value: Collaboration

Value: Education

Approach: Classroom accommodations

Value: Encouragement and support of first language use

Approach: Parent coaching

'Now I let him finish, even if it takes longer. I used to jump in. I didn't realize that was hurting more than helping,' Diego's mother reflects during the follow-up meeting.

Reflections

Diego's journey illuminates the profound intersection between trauma, identity, and communication. As a child who has already faced profound emotional adversity,

Diego's stuttering is not merely a matter of disrupted fluency—it is a visible manifestation of his internal struggle with safety, self-expression, and vulnerability. His disfluency increases not because he does not know what to say, but because saying it feels risky.

What became most evident throughout our sessions was that speech therapy could not occur in isolation from his emotional experience, which is why the therapeutic relationship must be established first. Only then could Diego begin to take the communicative risks that fluency therapy requires. He does not need to be 'fixed'; he needs to be heard, accepted, and empowered. One of the most impactful moments occurred when Diego began voluntarily raising his hand in class, using the strategies he learned in therapy and no longer fearing how others would react. Although his stuttering persists, his self-perception and communication confidence have significantly improved, which is a critical milestone.

Value: Therapeutic relationship

Diego's case reinforces that fluency is not the ultimate goal—communication is. Therapy must be personalized, culturally responsive, and sensitive to trauma histories. This distinction shapes my approach and guides my decision to include moments of emotional processing and mindfulness as integral parts of therapy. It also encourages close collaboration with school counselors, his parents, and teachers to create an environment that supports both his emotional and linguistic needs.

Value: Cultural responsiveness

Through Diego, the intervention team also learned the importance of embracing bilingualism not as a complication, but as a strength. Early in the process, there was concern that language switching might be worsening his stuttering, but further exploration revealed that Diego feels most at ease when he is allowed to use his full linguistic repertoire. Validating both English and Spanish in therapy gives him permission to be his whole self.

From a professional standpoint, this case taught me many key lessons, beginning with the importance of treating the whole child and not just their speech symptoms. In addition, the role of emotional safety and trust in communication should be recognized. I realize that trauma-informed care is not optional—it is essential when working with vulnerable populations, such as Diego. I must acknowledge that every child's communication profile is deeply personal, and that effective therapy must honor both the cognitive and emotional dimensions of speech. Furthermore, that progress is not always linear—some of Diego's greatest victories were internal shifts: increased self-acceptance, advocacy, and reduced avoidance. Bilingualism should not be seen as a clinical barrier, but instead, be celebrated and incorporated into treatment. I learned that the therapeutic relationship is just as important as the techniques used, and why collaborating with caregivers and other professionals is crucial for lasting progress. Most importantly, Diego reminds me that stuttering does not define a child—how they are supported does.

'*Thank you for helping me be brave with my words,*' Diego says during a therapy session.

Questions for reflection and discussion

1. What is the importance of conducting a comprehensive speech-language evaluation for a child referred for stuttering?
2. Why might it be appropriate for SLTs to use a trauma-informed approach with ALL clients who stutter?
3. What are some things an SLT can do to foster an open, safe, and welcoming therapeutic environment for a person who stutters?
4. What skills does an SLT need to establish a therapeutic relationship with a client?
5. How can an SLT support a client's bilingualism, even if the SLT does not speak the client's native language?
6. What are some ways to educate the public about stuttering to increase understanding and reduce the stigma that accompanies it?

Further reading

Chmela, K, & Reardon, N. (2001). ***The school-age child who stutters: Working effectively with attitudes and emotions.*** Stuttering Foundation of America.

International Stuttering Association: www.stutteringhelp.org/international-stuttering-association

Michael Palin Centre for Stammering. (n.d.). ***Michael Palin Centre for Stammering.*** Retrieved July 1, 2025, from https://michaelpalincentreforstammering.org/

Quesal, R. (2010). Empathy: Perhaps the most important E in EBP. ***Seminars in Speech and Language, 31***, 217–226.

Spero Stuttering: www.sperostuttering.org/

Further information

Theories

Adverse childhood experiences: are stressful and traumatic events experienced in childhood that are correlated with adverse outcomes throughout the lifespan for that individual. Research supports the link between early adverse experiences and later speech-language challenges (O'Leary et al., 2023).

Multifactorial causes of stuttering: there are multiple variables that contribute to the cause of stuttering, including motor, linguistic, and emotional factors (Smith & Weber, 2017).

Second language acquisition refers to the learning of a second language that is different from the individual's primary (or first) language. Second language acquisition can occur in a five-stage process, beginning with the preproduction stage, transitioning to early production, then speech emergence, followed with intermediate fluency, and completing with advanced fluency (Hyter & Salas-Provance, 2023).

Stuttering is a term reserved by speech-language clinicians to differentiate between instances of sensorimotor disruptions in the flow of speech with the hesitations and minor disfluencies observed in the typical daily speech of most people. The sensorimotor disruptions of stuttering include a loss of the capacity to control or regulate the speech actions that are necessary to move forward with the production of sounds or syllables (Yairi & Seery, 2023).

Approaches

Case history is an aspect of the assessment process that entails gathering as much background information as possible regarding the client who stutters. This information includes stuttering history, treatment history, current description of the speech problem, environmental variables affecting speech, impact of stuttering on quality of life, other relevant case history, and the client's perspective (Yairi & Seery, 2023).

Classroom accommodations, such as alternative methods for participation and extended response time, can be implemented to increase the academic success of a child who stutters.

Cognitive Behavioral Therapy (CBT) is a type of psychological therapy used to address anxiety and social withdrawal in children who stutter (Kelman & Wheeler, 2015).

Comprehensive speech-language assessment: in addition to the area of concern, a speech-language therapist should also assess all areas of speech and language to ensure that other problems do not exist that may be contributing to the main problem.

Consent to evaluate: a speech-language therapist must obtain written consent from the client or the client's guardian prior to conducting an assessment.

Group therapy: the advantages of group therapy include: 1) placing a group of people together with similar problems to provide comfort and support to each other; 2) providing a safe environment for the members to openly and honestly express themselves, provide feedback to each other, and allow the members to view their personal and social issues in a new perspective, and 3) facilitating the transfer of the strategies learned in individual therapy sessions by giving the group members opportunities to practice the learned speech patterns and behaviors with each other (Yairi & Seery, 2023).

Multi-disciplinary is the involvement of professionals from various disciplines (e.g., speech-language, psychology, counseling, social work, etc.) in the care of a client.

Parent coaching: for parents with a child who stutters, this entails showing them how to use wait time, active listening, and modeling calm speech, as well as encouraging them to reduce correction and interruption, and to use consistent emotional validation and patience with their child (Mumy, 2022).

The **Stuttering Severity Instrument (SSI-4)** is a valid and reliable normed-referenced stuttering assessment designed to assess and monitor stuttering severity in children and adults (Riley, 2009).

Stuttering therapy strategies: strategies aimed at producing deliberately fluent speech include slow and stretched speech, gentle voice initiated with airflow, light articulatory contact, and continuous articulatory movements. Strategies for the management of stuttering include pullout and cancellation procedures. Voluntary stuttering (also known as pseudostuttering) is intended to reduce avoidance and fear and build desensitization to feared speaking situations (Yairi & Seery, 2023).

Trauma-informed care is used to emphasize safety, consistency, and emotional regulation. In the practice of speech-language therapy, it entails maintaining a consistent routine across therapy sessions to reduce anxiety, providing visual schedules, and teaching the client mindfulness exercised to help them feel more in control and less threatened by communication demands (O'Leary et al., 2023).

Values

Acceptance: SLTs must not only demonstrate full respect and acceptance for their clients who stutter, whether they demonstrate stuttering behaviors, but also help them fully respect and accept themselves (Yairi & Seery, 2023).

Collaboration: entails the teamwork of the SLT with parents, teachers, counselors, psychologists, and other professionals to better serve the needs of a client.

Cultural responsiveness: used in assessment and treatment practices to accommodate the variability that exists in people from a variety of cultural and linguistic groups. This entails the conscious use of assessments and treatment materials that are as unbiased as possible and that take into consideration the unique capabilities found in diverse groups (Hyter & Salas-Provance, 2023).

Education: an SLT should provide information to parents, teachers, and others working with a child who stutters on the genetic and neurophysiological underpinnings of stuttering to increase understanding and empathy (Mumy, 2022).

Encouragement and support of first language use: the maintenance of a child's first language fosters confidence and language continuity (Mumy, 2022).

Therapeutic relationship is the relationship that the SLT should establish with a client prior to targeting intervention goals. This relationship must first become a place of trust, consistency, and safety.

References

Hyter, Y. D., & Salas-Provance, M. B. (2023). ***Culturally responsive practices in speech, language, and hearing sciences*** (2nd ed.). CA: Plural Publishing.

Kelman, E., & Wheeler, S. (2015). Cognitive behaviour therapy with children who stutter. ***Procedia – Social and Behavioral Sciences*, *193***, 165–174. https://doi.org/10.1016/j.sbspro.2015.03.255

Mumy, A. P. G. S. (2022). Culturally responsive guidelines for serving families of bilingual children who stutter. ***Perspectives of the ASHA Special Interest Groups*, *8***(1), 164–175. https://doi.org/10.1044/2022_persp-22-00004

O'Leary, N., Rupert, A. C., & Lotty, M. (2023). Understanding the why: The integration of trauma-informed care into speech and language therapy practice. ***Advances in Communication and Swallowing*, *26***(2), 81–87. https://doi.org/10.3233/ACS-230056

Riley, G. D. (2009). ***SSI-4: Stuttering Severity Instrument*** (4th ed.). Austin, TX: Pro-Ed.

Smith, A., & Weber, C. (2017). How stuttering develops: The multifactorial dynamic pathways theory. ***Journal of Speech, Language, and Hearing Research*, *60***(9), 2483–2505. https://doi.org/10.1044/2017_JSLHR-S-16-0343

Yairi, E., & Seery, C. H. (2023). ***Stuttering: Foundations and clinical applications*** (3rd ed.). San Diego, CA: Plural Publishing.

Case study 13
Kamila: differential diagnosis, different approaches or just differences?

Fernanda Dreux M. Fernandes

Kamila's history

Kamila was born in Kenya and is the only child of young parents. When Kamila was almost 3 years old the family moved to São Paulo in Brazil, following a job opportunity for her father at a university there. In Brazil, Kamila's mother opted not to work outside the home in order to spend as much time as possible with Kamila and to help her to adapt to her new surroundings. São Paulo is a very large and challenging city, so the family decided to live at a reasonable distance from the father's place of employment.

Four months after the move to São Paulo and at the beginning of the school year, Kamila was enrolled in the university's preschool. Her parents wanted her to have contact with other children and to learn Portuguese. This period coincided with the beginning of the university classes and Kamila started to be observed by students studying CSD (Communication Sciences and Disorders) and to participate in activities conducted by them. After a 3-month period, the students observed that Kamila had minimal interaction with her peers and spoke just a few words, some in English and some in what appeared to be Swahili. For example, she would say, *'want maji'*. We were able to verify that *'maji'* means *'water'* in Swahili. In discussion with their supervisor, the students referred Kamila to the CSD ambulatory service and was included in the Language Development Research Lab.

Theory: CSD (Communication Sciences and Disorders)

Theory: Language Development Research Lab

Setting

The university in which I work has a clinic that offers ambulatory services in speech-language pathology and in audiology as part of the supervised practice area of the

Theory: Phonoaudiliogy

DOI: 10.4324/9781003668756-17

Communication Sciences and Disorders programme in São Paulo, Brazil. Students gain experience in a wide range of practice settings covering a wide range of clinical presentations, working alongside graduate Phonoaudiologists. Students are supervised by a professor and researcher in the associated clinical area. The service is set up in such a way that it offers a wide range of opportunities for professional training to undergraduate students; clinical research and teaching; and supervision experiences to graduate students. As a publicly-funded university, it is a way for us to give back to the society, building knowledge that will improve the quality of the CSD practice based on data and results that refer to the Brazilian population. My role in the following scenario is as a clinical supervisor to CSD students working with Kamila and her family.

Meeting Kamila and her mother

Kamila is 3 years and 8 months old when the CSD students first meet her at the lab and under my supervision. Kamila's mother brings her to the appointment. The students begin by carrying out an initial interview with Kamila's mother. This is conducted in English. She appears shy and is unable to provide a lot of information about Kamila's development and routines.

The student begins by asking, *'What can you tell me about Kamila's development?'*

Kamila's mother responds, *'She grew up normal'*.

They ask a more targeted question, *'How old was she when she started to speak? Can you remember her first words?'*

Kamila's mother thinks for a moment before responding, *'she said mama, mother, and chupa, like...bottle...when she was a baby...'*

'Did she play with other children?', they ask.

Kamila's mother smiles, *'yes always running and laughing...'*

Value: Respect for diversity

Although some of the difficulties can be attributed to the fact that neither the students nor Kamila's mother are using their native languages, it seems she is not comfortable talking about her family and home, and this appears to be due to cultural differences. It is not possible to obtain any further background information from her at this stage. Kamila's father had been invited to attend the meeting as well but did not participate in this or any subsequent meeting or interview.

Following my interview, the students request that a basic audiology assessment is carried out with Kamila by the relevant CSD team. It shows that her hearing is within a normal range. Her overall behaviour has not raised any doubts about these results. The students assess her language in spontaneous play and Kamila is able to engage in non-verbal games and activities but she shows very little communicative initiative, largely following my lead. They assess her language more formally and this reveals she has a very limited vocabulary both in Portuguese and in English. It is difficult to maintain Kamila's attention and as such, no further meaningful results can be gained. For now, they conclude that she presents with a Language Development Disorder (LDD), and their main focus is to increase her vocabulary in order to improve her communication more generally. The students explain to Kamila's mother that they would like to enrol Kamila on a weekly language therapy programme with a focus on receptive and expressive vocabulary. The contents of this will be agreed in consultation with her preschool class teachers to ensure that the vocabulary is relevant to her current learning.

Theory: Language Development Disorder (LDD)

Approach: Vocabulary-based intervention

Social communication therapy for Kamila

After 3 months of therapy, Kamila is able to identify a large number of words in Portuguese and to name some everyday objects and activities. However, there is no increase in her initiating interactions or her engagement in games that involved the use of language.

The students decide to refer Kamila to another Research Lab, where the focus of language therapy will be on functional and pragmatic use of language. The approach chosen here is based around interactive play that encourages

Theory: Pragmatics

Value: Child-centered practice

Approach: Multi-modal communication

Approach: Involving parents

Value: Family empowerment

the use of verbal language. Sessions are taken at Kamila's pace, giving her time to process the situations and to express herself without pressure. Non-verbal communication is used to support Kamila's understanding and to enable her to express herself when she cannot find the words she wants to say. Kamila is encouraged to have an important role in choosing the toys and activities, and in controlling the overall pace of each session. Kamila's mother is actively involved in the therapy sessions too. This means she is able to observe her daughter playing and adopt new strategies to use with her at home. It also allows a space for her mother to express any concerns she has about Kamila's development. The idea in this setting is not to '*teach*' Kamila's mother, but rather to create situations where she can consider how her interactions could be improved at home.

Successful outcomes for Kamila

After 3 months of therapy, the students reassess Kamila. They video-record a short interaction between us and use this as the basis for analyzing her language. They observe significant improvements in a number of areas of her communication. Whereas previously, Kamila had been minimally communicative, she is now a more active participant in interactions. She is also able to initiate communication during play activities, for example, by suggesting the games she would like to play. She now uses non-verbal communication, such as pointing, gesture and facial expression alongside her verbal communication, and this shows she wants to be understood and is a sign of her improving social communication. Overall, these results are positive and suggest that this approach to therapy, focusing on Kamila's pragmatic skills through play, should continue.

Approach: Interdisciplinary referral

Kamila's mother also opens up to me now, expressing her difficulties in adapting to her new life in a different culture, with a different language and cultural expectations. She is thanked for being honest about these challenges and the students suggest referring her to the psychology service within the university. She agrees to this. In the following semester, the students meet Kamila and her mother again.

Both mother and daughter are now visibly more relaxed and able to enjoy each other's company more than before. For Kamila, she continues to show improvements in her interactions with others.

Reflections

For me, this case demonstrates how external factors in the child's environment can affect their development. Whilst working with Kamila and her mother, it became apparent that the child's speech and language difficulties were a *'warning flag'* for wider issues within the family. On the surface, the family's circumstances could be considered largely straight-forward. There were no legal issues in their move to a new country, since they were not refugees; there were no health or economic issues and they had a support network provided by the father's new job. Despite this, the adaptation to a new life was stressful for all and clearly impacted on Kamila at an important point in her development.

The process of moving from one country to the other can be challenging, even when it can be thought of as *'moving up'* or *'moving forward'*. Issues concerning living arrangements, including functional considerations (for example, where to shop; where to go for entertainment; access to doctors, dentists, hairdressers) can quickly add up and become stress factors. In this case, many of these issues were left to Kamila's mother to resolve. Indeed, it is not unusual that mothers may take on responsibility for aiding the whole family's adjustment to their new living arrangements. That is not to say that her father was absent, but rather that he had his own adaptations to make settling into a new job role in a new country.

In this case, Kamila's speech and language development difficulties were identified early and she was referred to a highly qualified service where the best approach could be offered. Instead of spending valuable time trying to determine one specific diagnosis, a short period of intervention was proposed to approach the most visible problem: Kamila's lack of knowledge and use of language. When it became clear that increasing the opportunity for acquiring

Value: Holistic support

new language was needed, the intervention focused on building communication interest and abilities. Involving Kamila's mother throughout her therapy ensured that her own doubts and concerns could be raised and solutions offered to address them – namely, the opportunity to use communication strategies with her daughter and access to psychology for her own personal needs.

Questions for reflection and discussion

1. What might it be like for families raising a child to transfer to different countries, with different languages and cultures, even when it may be an improvement in their lives?
2. What role should speech and language therapists play in identifying wider issues for families and providing support?
3. Is there a time limit for determining the need for changes in intervention procedures when progress is slower than expected?
4. What might be some of the limitations for diagnostic therapy with children?
5. What are the alternative solutions when the Phonoaudiologist (CSD professional) and the family (or the child) do not speak the same language?
6. How can the outcomes of the intervention process be assessed in a timely manner when working with a language that is not the child's first language?

Further reading

American Speech-Language-Hearing Association: www.ASHA.org

Clauss-Ehlers CS, Bela Sood A and Weist MD (Eds) (2020). ***Social Justice for Children and Young People – International Perspectives***. Cambridge University Press.

Fernandes FDM (Ed) (2017). ***Advances in Speech-Language Pathology***. IntechOpen.

Levey S, Moonsamy S (Eds) (2021) ***Unserved and Underserved Populations – New Approaches to Inclusivity***. Peter Lang Publishers

Misciagna S (Ed) (2020). ***Learning Disabilities – Neurological Bases, Clinical Features and Strategies of Intervention***. IntechOpen,

Further information

Theories

CSD (Communication Sciences and Disorders) is the overarching discipline in Brazil encompassing both the science of human communication and its disorders. It encapsulates the study of both Speech and Language Pathology and Audiology, enabling graduates to become Phonoaudiologists, which integrates the roles of the speech and language therapist and audiologist into a single profession.

Language Development Disorder (LDD), also referred to as Developmental Language Disorder (DLD), is a neurodevelopmental condition characterized by persistent difficulties in the comprehension and/or production of spoken language that cannot be attributed to intellectual disability, hearing loss, neurological damage, or inadequate exposure to language (Bishop et al., 2017).

Language Development Research Lab: research-led educational facilities in Brazil offering opportunities for supervised practice and clinical experience in different areas to students currently in different stages of professional training as Phonoaudiologists.

Phonoaudiliogy is the name of the discipline in Brazil that works with individuals who have speech, language, hearing, and swallowing difficulties.

Pragmatics relates to language use in real-life contexts and involves skills such as turn-taking, asking questions, or sharing feelings. It focuses on communication that has meaning in daily life (Ninio & Snow, 2018).

Approaches

Interdisciplinary referral is the practice of directing clients or families to other professionals when their needs go beyond a single field, ensuring holistic and coordinated care.

Involving parents in therapy offers them the opportunity to take an active role in their child's treatment, allowing them to observe, reflect, and apply communication strategies in the home environment.

Multi-modal communication is an approach that integrates verbal, non-verbal, and augmentative strategies to support expression and understanding, offering flexible and inclusive ways for individuals to communicate (Higham & Hebets, 2013).

Vocabulary-based intervention is a language therapy approach that promotes vocabulary acquisition by systematically teaching word meanings, semantic relationships, and functional use. It typically involves direct instruction, contextual embedding, strategy training, and technological support, thereby strengthening communication and supporting literacy development (Ansari et al., 2025).

Values

Child-centered practice is an approach that prioritizes children's interests, pace, and active participation in the therapeutic process, creating a supportive environment that fosters motivation, autonomy, and meaningful communication.

Family empowerment means helping parents feel more confident and capable of supporting their child, which is helpful in generalizing approaches used in the clinic to the child's wider communication environments.

Holistic support means caring not only for the child's language needs but also for the family's emotional and cultural well-being. Kamila's intervention supported both her communication and her mother's adaptation.

Respect for diversity means valuing different languages, cultures, and family roles. Kamila's mother's shyness and language barriers were seen as part of her cultural experience, not as deficits.

References

Ansari R, Chiat S, Cartwright M, Herman R. (2025). Vocabulary interventions for children with developmental language disorder: a systematic review. ***Frontiers in Psychology***. 16:1517311.

Bishop DV, Snowling MJ, Thompson PA, Greenhalgh T, Consortium C, Adams C, et al. (2017). Phase 2 of CATALISE: A multinational and multidisciplinary Delphi consensus study of problems with language development: Terminology. ***Journal of Child Psychology and Psychiatry***. 58(10):1068–80.

Higham JP, Hebets EA (2013). An introduction to multimodal communication. ***Behavioral Ecology and Sociobiology***. 67(9):1381–8.

Ninio A, Snow C. (2018). ***Pragmatic Development***. Routledge.

Case study 14
Bella: what next? A personal journey after a stroke

Neil Coull and Elissa Manzi

Bella's stroke and recovery

Bella was 79 when she had her stroke. She is now 81. Before her stroke, she lived an independent life with no significant health concerns. Her stroke has been a real shock to her, and she spent several months as an inpatient in hospital before being discharged home. She had a further eight months accessing community outpatient services, not only for Speech and Language Therapy but also Occupational and Physiotherapy. Her outpatient therapies have recently ended, and she has been discharged. Bella continues to have significant health challenges including mobility difficulties and aphasia. Combined, these difficulties mean that she is no longer able to enjoy the same social activities she enjoyed in the past, such as Zumba, painting, supporting children's reading in a local school and scrabble club. Bella continues to live alone but is finding her life increasingly lonely after her stroke.

Theory: Stroke

Approach: Neurorehabilitation

Theory: Aphasia

Meeting Bella

The first time I meet Bella is at a stroke group. It is run by volunteers, many of them having had strokes themselves in the past or who have been carers for family members who have had strokes. I offer occasional Speech and Language Therapy drop-in sessions there as part of my outreach role as a university lecturer. Bella has only recently joined the group as a way of meeting new people and, as she says, to give her *'something to do'*. The first time I see Bella, she is sitting alone. Volunteers at the group tell me that she rarely takes part in any of the group's activities and is often tearful. They say she does not seem to want to talk to anyone. I approach Bella:

Theory: Impact of stroke

DOI: 10.4324/9781003668756-18

'Hello, my name is Neil. I'm a Speech and Language Therapist. I wonder if I can have a chat with you?'. Bella nods and I pull up a chair.

'How are you today?', I ask. Bella smiles, rolls her eyes and shrugs.

It quickly becomes apparent that Bella has difficulties speaking due to aphasia.

'Can I ask some questions about your stroke and your communication?', I ask.

Bella has a puzzled look on her face. It appears that she does not understand everything that is said to her.

I take out pen and paper and write down *'stroke'*.

'You have had a stoke?' I ask with a deliberate inflection at the end of the sentence to indicate I am asking a question. Bella looks down at the page and nods.

I write down *'speech'*.

'You are having difficulties with speaking?' Bella nods, points to her mouth and shrugs.

Approach: Supported communication

We have a short conversation. I am mindful to ask one question or share one idea at a time. I write down key words, and if I am asking a question, I write down some choices. Bella responds well to this, largely using pointing, nodding and facial expression. I find out a bit about her life and her communication challenges.

Theory: Impact of aphasia on friendships

What becomes clear is that Bella's life has changed since her stroke. She is tearful when asked about friendships. It seems as though she is no longer able to do some of the things she enjoyed doing before. Using supported communication, Bella tells me that she lived an active life in the years since retiring with a wide group of friends and a range of interests. I ask about her friendships now and she looks sad. She tells me that some of her friends are no longer in touch with her since her stroke. She is unable to drive now, and it is hard for her to get on public transport due to difficulties walking now.

'*How did you get here today?*' I ask. Bella tries to say a word, but it is unclear.

'*Can you write down the word?*' I hand Bella a pen. She starts to write the letter T, then pauses and looks panicked.

'*Perhaps you could draw it*', I suggest. Bella draws the outline of a car.

'*Did someone drive you here?*', I ask. Bella nods.

I continue, '*Was it a friend or family member?*'. Bella looks a bit puzzled.

'*So, not a friend or family member*', I suggest. Bella shakes her head.

'*Was it a taxi?*' I ask. Bella nods.

Further conversation reveals that Bella's therapy recently ended. She feels sad about this, expressing that she feels hopeless for the future.

Approach: Discharge

Approach: Conversation Partners

Approach: Aphasia choirs

Before leaving the group, I share some leaflets with Bella about two initiatives that we offer through our university. The first is the Conversation Partners scheme. I explain to Bella that it is not therapy per se, but that she will have regular meetings with one of our Speech and Language Therapy students, and that they will have conversations together, very much as we are doing today. The second is an invitation to our aphasia choir. Bella is very keen on the idea of Conversation Partners. She is less sure about the choir, indicating that she will find it hard to sing. However, she agrees to go along and try it.

A year later...

I meet Bella again a year later at the same stroke group. When I arrive, she is proudly holding a scrap book with photographs and stories about her life which her Conversation Partner, Gemma, helped her to put together. Gemma is a student Speech and Language Therapist and has been visiting Bella as her Conversation Partner over the past six months. The volunteers at the stroke group comment that Bella appears much happier at the group now. Her aphasia has improved a little, but she still has difficulties expressing herself without using non-verbal communication, including writing, drawing and communication charts. Despite this, she is keen to chat to everyone in the group. She greets me with a beaming smile.

'And what about the choir?' I ask, *'are you still enjoying that?'*

Bella flicks through the pages of her scrap book landing on one with *'Choir'* written at the top of the page. There are photos of her and her new singing friends, and one of the photographs shows Bella and others performing in front of an audience of friends and family with the caption, *'Christmas Concert'*.

I ask Bella how things are now, and she smiles and points to the photograph of her new friends at the choir.

Moving on with life and living well with aphasia

Two years after her stroke, Bella continues to have significant difficulties with aphasia. Despite this, her confidence has grown in her abilities as a communicator. She uses lots of different ways to express herself, including writing and drawing, and a life book that her student Conversation Partner created with her. She now has a rich social life with new friends and a newfound love of singing. Bella recently signed up to become a Conversation Partners trainer. This means that she will support the development of students, like Gemma, to learn skills in supported communication so that they can go out and make a difference, as Gemma did for Bella. Ultimately, the role of the Speech and Language Therapist in this situation is to enable someone to live well with aphasia, by helping them to identify relevant and fulfilling activities and support them to take part in these.

Reflections

There is a role for Speech and Language Therapists to think beyond the clinic. In this case, I was able to signpost Bella to initiatives within our own department: a Conversation Partners scheme and our aphasia choir. Bella seemed to gain a great deal from both. They gave her a new sense of purpose, greater confidence in her communicative abilities and offered her a chance to make new friends. Whilst neither looks like therapy in the traditional clinical sense, both initiatives offer opportunities to develop communication skills in everyday activities, namely, having a conversation and participating in social activities with others. Unfortunately, the availability of such initiatives is somewhat limited by location. It is hoped that through research into these types of activity, they will become more prevalent. Introducing them to university students studying Speech and Language Therapy will hopefully inspire them to develop these types of longer-term interventions in their own future careers.

Bella appeared to gain a lot of confidence from taking part in the Conversation Partners scheme. Her student Conversation Partner, Gemma, was mindful of her own communication. For example, she discovered that Bella was often more successful responding to closed questions than open questions. A closed question tends to have a small and limited range of answers (such as yes or no). It also became apparent that Bella was able to draw successfully when she got stuck for words. Sometimes, she could write down parts of the word she was trying to find. Gemma made sure that there was always pen and paper to hand during her visits. She also came to the meetings prepared with a folder of resources, including maps and images of different everyday topics related to Bella's hobbies. Sometimes these images were helpful if Bella was unable to find the word she was looking for.

Value: Accessible communication

The impact of music on aphasia recovery has been explored in literature. Listening to music daily has been shown to improve post-stroke language recovery (Sihvonen et al., 2021). It is common for people with aphasia to retain their ability to sing or hum a melody. Research suggests that singing can result in structural neuroplasticity changes in left frontal language areas and bilateral language pathway, even for those with chronic aphasia (Sihvonen et al., 2024). It can also increase individual wellbeing and foster a sense of community (Tamplin et al., 2013).

Although she was initially reluctant to join the choir because of her aphasia, the Conversation Partners scheme gave her the confidence to go along and meet new people. At first, attending the aphasia choir made her nervous – words didn't come easily, and she feared being misunderstood. But as the group sang together, something shifted; the rhythm and melody helped the words flow more freely. There was no pressure to join in, but Bella recognised many of the songs and they evoked different memories and emotions. Surrounded by others who shared similar challenges, she felt understood, supported and proud to use her voice.

Questions for reflection and discussion

1. In what ways do you think the communication and physical difficulties associated with a stroke could impact on individuals' lives?
2. Why do you think that a person's social circles might decrease as the result of a stroke?
3. Why might a person's mood change following a stroke?
4. How can Speech and Language Therapists support psychological adjustment to stroke and aphasia?
5. How can Speech and Language Therapists promote 'living well with aphasia'?
6. What types of initiatives or activities might be helpful to individuals post-stroke to help them connect with others and improve their quality of life?

Further reading

Aphasia Reconnect: https://aphasiareconnect.org/

Better Conversations with Aphasia: An E-learning Resource: www.ucl.ac.uk/short-courses/search-courses/better-conversations-aphasia-e-learning-resource

Chapey, R. (Ed.) (2008), ***Language intervention strategies in aphasia and related neurogenic communication disorders***. Philadelphia: Lippincott, Williams and Williams

Pound, C., Parr, S., Lindsay, J., & Woolf, C. (2000). ***Beyond Aphasia.*** Oxford: Routledge.

Stroke Association – Communication tools for aphasia: www.stroke.org.uk/stroke/effects/aphasia/communication-tools

Further information

Theories

Aphasia: an impairment to the language centres of the brain, typically as a result of acquired brain injury. Individuals with aphasia may experience challenges in producing language through speaking and writing, or understanding others through verbal and written messages.

Impact of aphasia on friendships: communication breakdowns caused by aphasia can lead to frustrations for the individual but also for those around them. As a result, friendships can deteriorate, often because of feelings of awkwardness or embarrassment or a lack of understanding of aphasia and how to support communication (Azios et al., 2022).

Impact of stroke: strokes can have life-changing effects on individuals including altered life goals and changes in employment and social activities (Bright et al., 2020).

Stroke: causes a suspension of blood flow to the brain which can result in neurological damage (Grefkes & Fink, 2020).

Approaches

Aphasia choirs provide a unique and uplifting way for people with aphasia to reconnect with language, music and each other. Singing engages different parts of the brain than speaking, often making it easier for participants to express themselves and communicate.

Conversation Partners is a form of social intervention that pairs up people with aphasia with communication partners who are skilled in supported conversation. As such, the purpose of Conversation Partners is not to directly treat communication impairments, but rather to provide enjoyable social opportunities for individuals with aphasia and practice in using different methods of communication (Horton et al., 2020).

Discharge from healthcare services can be challenging for many individuals post-stroke, particularly if they have not returned to the same level of functioning as they were before their stroke. Recovery from stroke can be slow and many individuals with aphasia may have chronic or long-lasting communication difficulties (Royal College of Speech and Language Therapists [RCSLT], 2025).

Neurorehabilitation: treatment often involves partnership working between numerous medical and healthcare professionals due to the complex patterns of impairment resulting from stroke.

Supported communication: people with aphasia are often very good communicators, despite their difficulties processing language. Supported conversation approaches focus on the person's existing communication skills rather than their difficulties. Supported communication techniques include providing information in other forms as well as speech, such as writing down words, using images and gesture (Pound et al., 2000).

Values

Accessible communication: ensuring the accessibility of communication is a core concern of all healthcare professionals, regardless of whether individuals have specific communication difficulties (Health and Care Professions Council [HCPC], 2025).

References

Azios, J. H., Strong, K. A., Archer, B., Douglas, N. F., Simmons-Mackie, N., & Worrall, L. (2022). Friendship matters: A research agenda for aphasia. ***Aphasiology*, *36***(3), 317–336. https://doi.org/10.1080/02687038.2021.1873908

Bright, F. A. S., McCann, C. M., & Kayes, N. M. (2020). Recalibrating hope: A longitudinal study of the experiences of people with aphasia after stroke. ***Scandinavian Journal of Caring Sciences*, *34***(2), 428–435. https://doi.org/10.1111/scs.12745

Grefkes, C., & Fink, G. R. (2020). Recovery from stroke: Current concepts and future perspectives. ***Neurological Research & Practice*, *2***(16), 1–10. https://doi.org/10.1186/s42466-020-00060-6

Health and Care Professions Council (HCPC). (2025). ***Standards of conduct, performance and ethics: Communication***. www.hcpc-uk.org/standards/standards-of-conduct-performance-and-ethics/revised-standards/communication/

Horton, S., Humby, K., & Jerosch-Herold, C. (2020). Development and preliminary validation of a patient-reported outcome measure for conversation partner schemes: The Conversation and Communication Questionnaire for People with Aphasia (CCQA). ***Aphasiology*, *34***(9), 1112–1137. https://doi.org/10.1080/02687038.2019.1700991

Kübler-Ross, E. (1969). ***On death and dying***. New York: Macmillan.

Pound, C., Parr, S., Lindsay, J., & Woolf, C. (2000). ***Beyond aphasia: Therapies for living with communication disability***. Routledge.

Royal College of Speech and Language Therapists (RCSLT). (2025). ***Aphasia overview***. www.rcslt.org/speech-and-language-therapy/clinical-information/aphasia/

Sihvonen, A. J., Pitkäniemi, A., Siponkoski, S. T., Kuusela, L., Martínez-Molina, N., Laitinen, S., Särkämö, E. R., Pekkola, J., Melkas, S., Schlaug, G., Sairanen, V., & Särkämö, T. (2024). Structural neuroplasticity effects of singing in chronic aphasia. ***eNeuro*, *11***(5), 1–15. https://doi.org/10.1523/ENEURO.0408-23.2024

Sihvonen, A. J., Ripollés, P., Leo, V., Saunavaara, J., Parkkola, R., Rodríguez-Fornells, A., Soinila, S., & Särkämö, T. (2021). Vocal music listening enhances post-stroke language network reorganization. ***eNeuro*, *8***(4), 1–15. https://doi.org/10.1523/ENEURO.0158-21.2021

Tamplin, J., Baker, F. A., Jones, B., Way, A., & Lee, S. (2013). Stroke a chord: The effect of singing in a community choir on mood and social engagement for people living with aphasia after stroke. ***NeuroRehabilitation*, *32***(4), 929–941. https://doi.org/10.3233/NRE-130916

Conclusion

Maria Garraffa

Speech and Language Therapy (SLT) is wide-reaching, and the cases presented in this book demonstrate how the profession can enhance the lives of those facing challenges with communication and swallowing across the lifespan of all areas of society. As has been demonstrated in the case studies, the role of the SLT involves complex decision making to address a wide array of clinical scenarios, considering the needs, hopes, and expectations of individuals whilst also adhering to the research evidence base.

The world does not remain static with society changing and the evidence base itself evolving. As such, SLTs must keep abreast of the latest research whilst also developing their practical skills in delivering interventions and their interpersonal skills in responding to the various needs of a range of stakeholders, including individual service users, their family members, friends, carers and other healthcare professionals. The future of SLT faces a complex mix of challenges and opportunities. Rapid demographic shifts, displacement, technological innovation, and rising expectations are all changing the landscape of communication disorders. Key among the challenges is an increased movement of people, through migration, displacement, and conflict zones; an ageing population; and the accelerating effects of digitalisation on communication. Yet these same forces also offer openings for more inclusive, flexible, culturally aware, and technologically enhanced practice. Drawing together what is known, and pointing to where experience must inform tomorrow's SLT, shows that observational skills, cultural humility, and learning across borders and professions will be essential.

Having read the complexity of the case studies presented in this book, we should embrace the SLT profession as active agents of our own professional development. Key attributes of this include self-efficacy, reflection, and a willingness to learn and develop.

The theory of self-efficacy proposed by Bandura (1997) is a good tool to frame how to use this book and support self-reflection on the decision-making processes needed in SLT practice. Within this theory is a belief in one's own ability to succeed and the motivation to develop. SLTs must be primed to develop through learning from themselves and others, and by honest reflection to master their skills and decision-making abilities. A core belief in one's ability to succeed is key to becoming a skilled SLT. That belief grows through experience. Confidence is built through professionals' reflections on their actions and impact by trying therapy techniques themselves and seeing that they work, turning each success into proof of growing ability. Watching experienced therapists and classmates work with clients can be inspiring. Encouragement and feedback from supervisors, mentors, and peers also shape how capable you feel—praise can lift your confidence, while constructive criticism helps you grow. Even your emotions play a part: feeling calm and focused can boost your belief in yourself, while nerves can make you doubt your skills. Together, these experiences shape your self-efficacy, helping you become more confident, capable, and ready to support the people you will work with in the future.

Considering future developments, a significant challenge for the SLT profession is migration and multilingualism. Therapists increasingly work with children and adults whose home language(s) differ from the majority or societal language (Pert, 2022). This raises issues of diagnostic accuracy, late referrals, misidentification of language differences as disorders (and vice versa), as well as lack of appropriately normed tools in the heritage languages. Similarly, the cultural views of disability and communication differ; what is considered acceptable in one cultural context may differ in another, including expectations about speech clarity, use of silence, roles of elders, or style of storytelling. Interpreters can help, but their role is made more difficult when subtleties of pragmatic, non-verbal communication or cultural nuances are involved.

An ageing population introduces its own set of challenges. Many older people will experience acquired communication disorders: age-related hearing loss, cognitive-communication problems (for example, from mild cognitive impairment or dementia), stroke-related aphasia, or motor speech issues like dysarthria or dysphagia. Their needs are often under recognised or undervalued; access to services, digital literacy, and physical or cognitive barriers may impede uptake. This means SLT services must adapt both in how they deliver services (e.g. flexibility, tele practice, in-home) and in terms of tools and interfaces (large fonts, simpler navigation, more support).

Children living in conflict zones or displaced by war pose a particularly severe set of challenges; a domain still not covered in language and communication disorders. They often endure trauma, disruptions of schooling, loss of caregivers, nutritional and health deficits, hearing-loss risk from injury or lack of healthcare access, unstable environments, and unsupported language learning (moving across linguistic communities, loss of exposure to one or more languages, perhaps inconsistent input). These children may also have less access to trained clinicians, reliable assessment tools, or intervention services. The mental health burden is high, compounding communication delays or impairments. Though the literature is less extensive here than for other populations, we know that for such children, early intervention is especially critical, but also hardest to deliver.

Digitalisation and technology offer huge opportunities still to be clarified and consistently included in the practice. The COVID-19 pandemic forced many SLTs to adopt remote working, tele practice, virtual assessment, and intervention tools. Technology—apps, automated screening tools, augmentative and alternative communication (AAC), social robots, interactive games—offers potential for scalable interventions, therapy in homes or schools that lack local specialists, greater interactivity, and increased engagement. But risks include digital divides (not everybody has access to stable internet, appropriate devices, privacy, trained caregivers), questions about fidelity and efficacy compared to face-to-face therapy, loss of non-verbal cues, or overreliance on technology at the expense of human relational components. Also, there are ethical issues around data privacy, cultural appropriateness of software or AI models, language bias in recognition systems, and potential exclusion of those with complex needs.

Another challenge cuts across all these issues: resource constraints, workforce shortages, uneven geographical distribution of clinicians, access inequalities tied to socioeconomic status, cultural or language minority status. SLT services in many low- and middle-income countries, and even in underserved communities within high-income countries, are under-resourced (Marshall et al., 2024). Early detection and preventive interventions are often limited; waiting times are long; children or adults may never receive services. Mental health, educational, and social consequences ensue. The UK, for instance, has had reports of many children with speech and language needs, many waiting long periods for therapy, with schools and parents reporting negative outcomes on attendance, academic participation, friendships, and mental health.

Yet there are many opportunities. Migration and multilingualism can enrich practice: therapists who learn new languages or partner with bilingual practitioners, interpreters, and community resources can develop more inclusive, culturally responsive approaches. Training curricula can incorporate multilingual norms, heritage language assessment, cross-linguistic variation, and cultural competence. In some places, AAC and technology can allow people with severe communication disorders to participate more fully in digital and social life. The demand for such tools may drive innovation.

Ageing populations can foster the growth of SLT specialisms in geriatric communication, cognitive-communication disorders, rehabilitation after neurological disease; also, preventive strategies to promote communication health across lifespan (e.g. hearing screening, public health campaigns, caregiver training, community-based interventions). Digital tools can support older adults through tele-practice, remote monitoring, hearing assistive tech, smart devices, voice-activated systems, even socially assistive robots. When designed well, these technologies can help mitigate some issues of mobility, isolation, or scarcity of clinicians in remote areas.

In conflict or displaced settings, mobile clinics, teletherapy across borders, partnerships with NGOs, schools, and community training (lay health workers, teachers) can be leveraged. Technology can help here too: remote training of local paraprofessionals, apps to support language exposure, digital audio libraries, translation tools—all of which have been used in humanitarian settings.

On digitalisation: blended service models combine in-person and remote aspects, flexible scheduling, parent or caregiver mediated therapy, online peer groups, virtual reality or augmented reality environments. Research into AI tools, ASR, and automated screening show promise—if backed by rigorous evaluation, culturally unbiased training data, accessible design, and ethical deployment.

In conclusion, as SLT practice enters this changing world, learning from experience will become even more critical. Therapists will need sharper observational skills: watching not only for speech errors or delayed milestones, but for how culture, social context, multilingual exposure, trauma, digital environments, and ageing affect communication. They must observe how clients use language in different settings—home, school, being online, and across cultures. Simultaneously, SLTs must engage in shared learning: from colleagues in other cultures, research in low- and middle-income countries, refugee and migrant communities, older populations, technologists designing AI tools, and families themselves. Therefore, the future depends not merely on technologies or demographic pressures, but on our ability to learn through observation, to adapt flexibly across different contexts, to share across cultures and disciplines, and to build SLT practice that is rooted in both evidence and empathy.

References

Bandura, A. (1997). ***Self-efficacy: The exercise of control***. Freeman.

Marshall, J., Wylie, K., McLeod, S., et al. (2024). Communication disability in low and middle-income countries: a call to action. ***BMJ Glob Health***, 9: e015289. doi:10.1136/bmjgh-2024-015289

Pert, S. (2022). ***Working with children experiencing speech and language disorders in a bilingual context: a home language approach***. Routledge.

Index

For Product Safety Concerns and Information please contact our
EU representative GPSR@taylorandfrancis.com Taylor & Francis
Verlag GmbH, Kaufingerstraße 24, 80331 München, Germany